Silenced by the WEIGHT of the Matriarchal Crown

# Arts, Creativities, and Learning Environments in Global Perspectives

*Series Editors*

Tatiana Chemi (*Aalborg University*)
Anu M. Mitra (*Union Institute & University*)

VOLUME 14

The titles published in this series are listed at *brill.com/acle*

# Silenced by the WEIGHT of the Matriarchal Crown

*A Baby Boomer Speaks about Becoming Anorexic*

*By*

Dicki Johnson Macy

BRILL

LEIDEN | BOSTON

Cover illustration: Photograph by Dicki Johnson Macy

All chapters in this book have undergone peer review.

The Library of Congress Cataloging-in-Publication Data is available online at https://catalog.loc.gov

Typeface for the Latin, Greek, and Cyrillic scripts: "Brill". See and download: brill.com/brill-typeface.

ISSN 2589-9813
ISBN 978-90-04-71103-7 (paperback)
ISBN 978-90-04-71104-4 (hardback)
ISBN 978-90-04-71105-1 (e-book)
DOI 10.1163/9789004711051



This book is printed on acid-free paper and produced in a sustainable manner.

# Contents

PREFACE

# Symbology of the Title—Who Decides What Is Real?

The origin of the word *real,* in English, stems from the word which means r*egal* or pertaining to the *King.* The ideal King reigns over everything as far as the eye can see. What he cannot see is not royal, is not real (Frye, 1983, p. 155), and is therefore disregarded or made invisible. Reality is that which pertains to the one in power. In a patriarchal society, the father's society, he, the King, has the power. He determines what is real and what is worthy of being heard or seen. His design prevails. Her crown, mother's crown, is designed by the King.

The metaphorical *Matriarchal or Maternal Crown,* in my title, symbolized her, the Queen's, adornment: her costume's head dress. She is beautifully clad for her role in the patriarch's theatre. Symbolic of her submission to his dominance, she concedes to his life of royalty. She understands that she is his jewel; She exists to shine light on her King. And she will pass her crown down to her chosen female progeny, her Princess. She will fashion her daughter's crown after her own image. For her King, she upholds the maintenance of her crown, daily polishing it to magnificence. Dazzling but heavy is this crown. Its weight, overtime, muffles her voice. Silent, her truths concealed, she finds belonging in his kingdom.

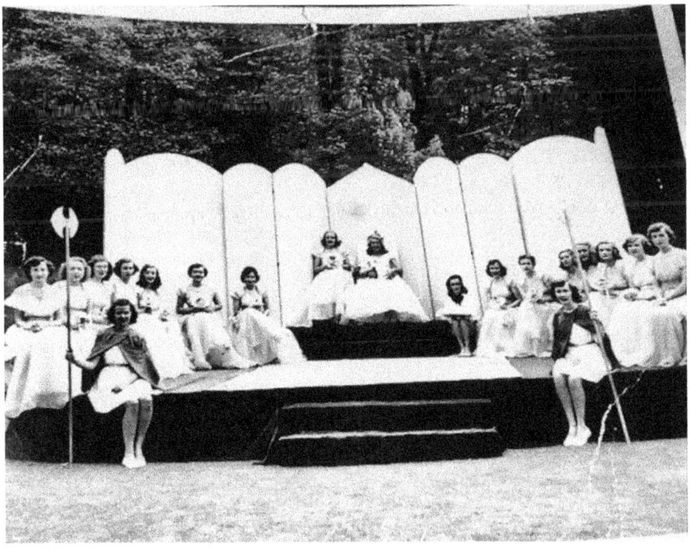

FIGURE P.1 Mom's Cotillion Ceremony, 1947

## Acknowledgements

You, because you love me, have listened patiently to my words.

You have responded with the affirmations that gave me the courage to tell my story to strangers.

Words can never express the gratitude which I extend to you, my family: Pompi, Dylan, Nina, Jade and to my mentors Jeanne, Jared, and Anu.

# Figures

# Introduction

> Silence is the ocean of the unsaid, the unspeakable, the repressed, the erased, the unheard. It surrounds the scattered islands made up of those allowed to speak and of what can be said and who listens.
>
> REBECCA SOLNIT (2017)

∴

When I was fourteen, I stopped eating, and nobody asked me why.

Then, as a fourteen-year-old girl, I didn't think much about not being asked. Now, as the adult woman looking back, I am stunned by the recollection. Then, I was rarely asked what I thought about or what motivated me. Rather, I was expected to excel, without questioning, at being the perfect student, daughter, and developing female person.

During my childhood I seemed to be unaware of any misfortune or irregularity with the adult world's lack of interest in my opinions. I remember feeling as if I was constantly floating, as if I were being carried forward without much thought to where I was going or who was steering the wheel. Carol Gilligan (2023) in her study of girls, puts words to my experience:

> I became a witness to dissociation-and to a not knowing that was culturally inscribed and socially enforced. Yet what I learned to think of as steps in a developmental progression, the separation of reason from emotion, of the mind from the body, and the self from relationships milestones on the march towards rationality, autonomy, immaturity held this not knowing in place. (p. 29)

Where was my voice, my place at the wheel? I was thinking that if my voice was a song, it would be a duet, or maybe a fugue composed[1] from the notes of my dyadic beginnings, with my mother, with my father. I looked back and saw a very different "me" in the lives I shared with each. I remember the beginnings.

> We usually recognize the beginning. Endings are more difficult to detect. Most often they are realized only after reflection. *Silence.* We are seldom conscious when silence begins—it is only afterwards that we realize what we have been a part of. (Williams, 2001, p. 193)

 | DOI:10.1163/9789004711051_001

I was silent in the physical duality of my existence: In my mother's home, I was a child prematurely groomed to be an adult; In my father's home, my childhood was sustained. This polarity amplified the conflictual sense of identity which clouded my coming of age. I was in training to be a woman. In the patriarchal society I would be bilingual: My silenced voice, my native tongue, held my intuition, my life experiences, and unique power. My scripted Female voice, my second language, alone was I allowed to speak. Survival in *his* world meant playing the scripted roles in the theatre of dominance and subordination. Yet my native tongue has not been forgotten. Today I question how the two voices might become harmonious, and in that harmony find empowerment. There are jewels found in the symbolic space between the inhale and the exhale, the bridge of negotiating balance and integrating the two. As Shinoda Bolen (2014) observes: "I see every woman as a woman in between acted on from within by goddess archetypes (powerful inner forces) and from without by cultural stereotypes" (p. 4).

Social and political discourses brandish competitive agendas; parents, teachers, clergy, political figures, and the media are diverse in their teaching. Looking for guidance, girls find themselves lost in a sea of mixed messages. Coming of age in a chaotic world, these girls attempt to fashion their identity and to find a place of belonging. In the chaos, they look and listen for one consistent message, one that speaks of safety and truth. In the patriarchy, this message does not exist. In the patriarchy voices compete rather than commune. It is within this culture that I sought to find my teenaged female self. This book is the story of that desperate journey and of my arts-based healing process.

This book draws attention to the patriarchal mandates placed upon women during the 1960s. It also explores the impacts which the media and the maternal relationship have upon this adolescent girl's developing sense of identity. The impact of the media, in all its expressions (film, music, stories, art) was and still is, both subliminal and profound. I suggest that the 1960s media supported the patriarchal scripts designed to subordinate women. I also posit that my own identity was directly impacted by my mother's relationship to the 1950s (post-World War Two) female script. I have recognized that my mother, as a daughter, had been a victim of this unhealthy scripting, and she too had suffered from a lack of secure attachment and maternal nurturing. "Mothers have a right to their anguish, to their conflict, to their doubt and ambivalence and uncertainty about their roles. Why should a woman because she gives birth to a child, ceased to be troubled by the profound social and cultural and existential questions?" (Chernin, 1985, p. 73). I do not want to throw my mother under the metaphorical bus, but rather to acknowledge that she too had been a generational victim of the patriarchy.

This book is an offering to women of all ages, to caregivers, clinicians and to mothers; It is an offering that might assist each in achieving or seeking out the before suggested harmony. It is an offering to girls who have been denied rituals and rites of passage into womanhood. It is an offering to all women whose lived experiences and intuitive knowledge have been devalued. I have created and offer examples of rituals and practices for self-discovery and for validating group development.

I share my memories of the female suppression which I experienced as a girl growing up in 1960s America. The writing of this book has given me the platform, the permission, and the support to ask *myself* the question, "Why did you stop eating", and perhaps, "why do other 14-year-olds stop eating?"

Find within this volume two distinct books: Part 1 is my memoir ("She Speaks"); Part 2 ("They Speak") sets the stage for exploring female identity development, highlighting historical, psychological, and social influences. You the reader, may choose to first immerse yourself in the narrative (Part 1) or to stand back and get an overview (Part 1), prior to that immersion.

My memoir traces the loss of my voice, the metaphorical *singing voice* that I equate with belonging. I have limited the memories to those prior to high school, to the foundations for my coming-of-age choices. I share the discovery of my authentic voice, which had been silenced by the scripted one. I am hopeful that in hearing my voice, others will find the courage to act and to question rather than lying in impotent wait for someone else's answers. As the elder poet Rilke (1934) stated to his young protégé: "Live the questions now. Perhaps you will then gradually, without noticing it, live along some distant day into the answer" (p. 35). I, like the elder poet, offer my narrative, to mothers and to young girls. I hope to lead by example rather than by coercion. My story is one in which I chose to express my voice through the vocal body; I chose Anorexia.

## Note

1 A contrapuntal composition in which a short melody or phrase (the subject) is introduced by one part and successively taken up by others and developed by interweaving the parts. Also a state or period of loss of awareness of one's identity, often coupled with flight from one's usual environment, associated with certain forms of hysteria and epilepsy (retrieved from Oxford Dictionary).

## References

Chernin, K. (1985). *The hungry self: Women, eating and identity*. HarperCollins.

Gilligan, C. (2023). *In a human voice*. Harvard University Press.

Rilke, R. M. (1934). *Letters to a poet as a young man.* W.W. Norton & Co. Inc.

Solnit, R. (2017). *The mother of all questions.* Haymarket Books.

Williams, T. T. (2001). *Refuge.* Vintage Books.

Williams, T. T. (2001). Why I write. In C. Force & P. Gerard (Eds.), *Writing creative non-fiction.* F.W. Publications.

# PART 1

## *She Speaks*

CHAPTER 1

# Introduction: Memoir Snapshots

> Memory… defines, creates, and holds a person's mental world together.
>
> LEWIS ET AL. (2001, p. 101)

∴

**snapshot**

*noun*

an informal photograph, especially one taken quickly by a handheld camera.

*Hunting*. a quick shot taken without deliberate aim.

*Informal*. a brief look, summary, or profile.

*Computing*: a record of the contents of a storage location or data file at a given time[1]

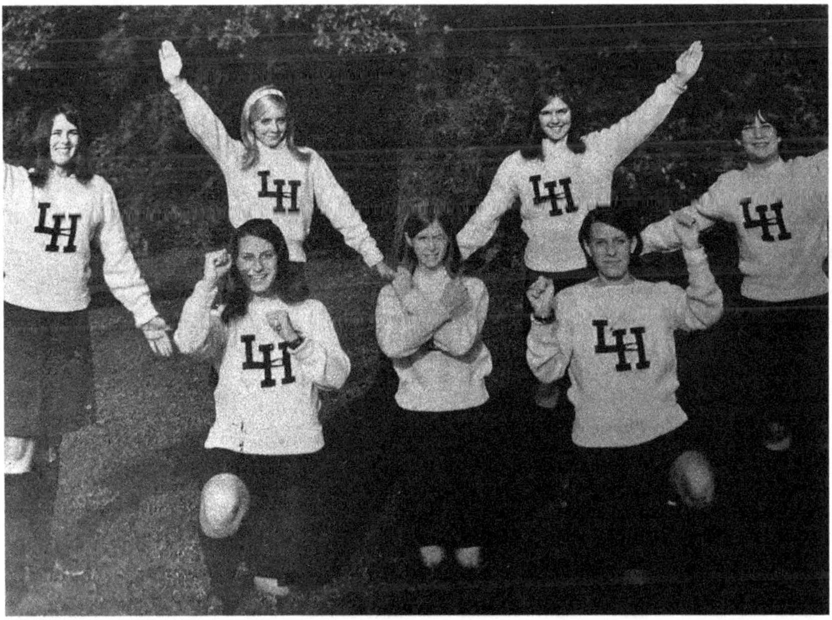


FIGURE 1 The author, cheerleader, center stage, 1967

 | DOI:10.1163/9789004711051_002

*Snapshot* well describes, in all its aberrations, the structure and formatting of my memoir selections. Each of these snapshots is short, informal, and quick. Each offers a brief look into my childhood and into my coming-of-age without following a chronological progression. The sequencing meanders through time, as do the memories that surface and beg to be noticed. I have limited each to approximately five hundred words. I have deliberately limited the time frame from which they have been extrapolated, to my first sixteen years of life. This time frame represents the prelude to my Anorexia.

My first snapshot, coincidentally, includes the remembrance of a battlefield. Hunting and the shooting of guns was the original referent for the word *snapshot.* A metaphorical battlefield, a warfare between discordant and conflictual voices, describes the landscape of my social and political childhood. It was not until 1900[2] that the word became associated with photography. Synchronicity. Photographs are center stage in this memoir. They have been catalysts for the recovering of my stories. They have also been characters in the theatre of my childhood. Taking photographs of one another gave me and my siblings a vehicle for conversation. Our voices, once muted, became visual voices. We spoke to each other in pictures.

## 1 Red

Our first air-conditioned car arrived new, joining our family like its seventh child. She was the only one that was not a blond child. She did not follow my mother's palette of powder blue and white. She was proud to be black, with red leather interior. My divorced father owned a Chevrolet and Cadillac dealership. My mother reaped the benefit of the "family discount" even though Mom wasn't his wife anymore. A floor model and the first with air-conditioning, she was the best choice for our annual family trip, despite her color.

Every year we ventured, all eight of us, to historical sites which my mother chose for us to explore. Worthwhile to mention, Mom also had a new toy for this trip. The super eight movie camera was firmly affixed to her face, an appendage that gave her an excuse to only look straight ahead. We six children were always at her periphery.

My stepfather Tom, whom we called Daddy, was always the designated driver. Three of us sat in the second seat, with the three youngest of us in the smaller third, back seat. My place was right behind Daddy's. My vista was either the back of his head or whatever I saw travel by to my left, as I gazed out of that window. Of course, the windows were closed throughout the trip as we were not to miss the airconditioned experience, despite the cost to run it. We were headed for Gettysburg, Pennsylvania the site of many bloody Civil War battles. The battle site "adventures" were long, hot, and tedious because Mom felt it important to film each word etched into each monument:

> The Battle of Gettysburg, fought from July 1 to July 3, 1863, is considered the most important engagement of the American Civil War. After a great victory over Union forces at Chancellorsville, General Robert E. Lee marched his Army of Northern Virginia into Pennsylvania in late June 1863.

## 2 Maternity

Mom is standing over my poodle, Mitzi who is in labor, super eight movie camera in hand. My young siblings, all six of them, hover over Mom, attempting to see the new pup as it emerges from the darkness of Mitzi's body. Mom lifts the laboring dog's leg, bringing light to the opening. I am thinking, even as a 12-year-old, that this intimate moment has been unjustly invaded. Mom seems obsessed with filming every beginning. I wonder why it is she never films *us* doing our regular everyday things. I know, even then, that Mom has never been keen on the long journey. She has always been a sprinter.

Making babies came easy to her. In all, she had ten pregnancies. She lost a son before me, twins between Ann and Tommy, and another boy the year before Billy. As a mother to infants, she was the Queen. She seemed to lose interest when they learned to walk and talk, when they started to ask questions that demanded a different kind of attention. So, as the eldest, I was anointed with the Princess crown. It became my job to attend to her animated but needy flock.

Yet Mom was generous. She loved animals and always had as many of them as she had children. Two horses, three dogs, and two cats. As you will remember, she loved beginnings and didn't seem to have the interest, or foresight, perhaps to imaging what future would flow from each of her beginnings. She was a lover of the moment. So, each Easter she gifted each of her seven children with special gifts from the Easter Bunny. One year we received seven adorable baby yellow chicks. Another, seven tiny white bunnies. Her gift-giving made Easter mornings were so exciting. The problem was that she didn't prepare for little yellow chicks growing to be big chickens, or little white bunnies to large rabbits. I can't remember what became of the chickens, but I do

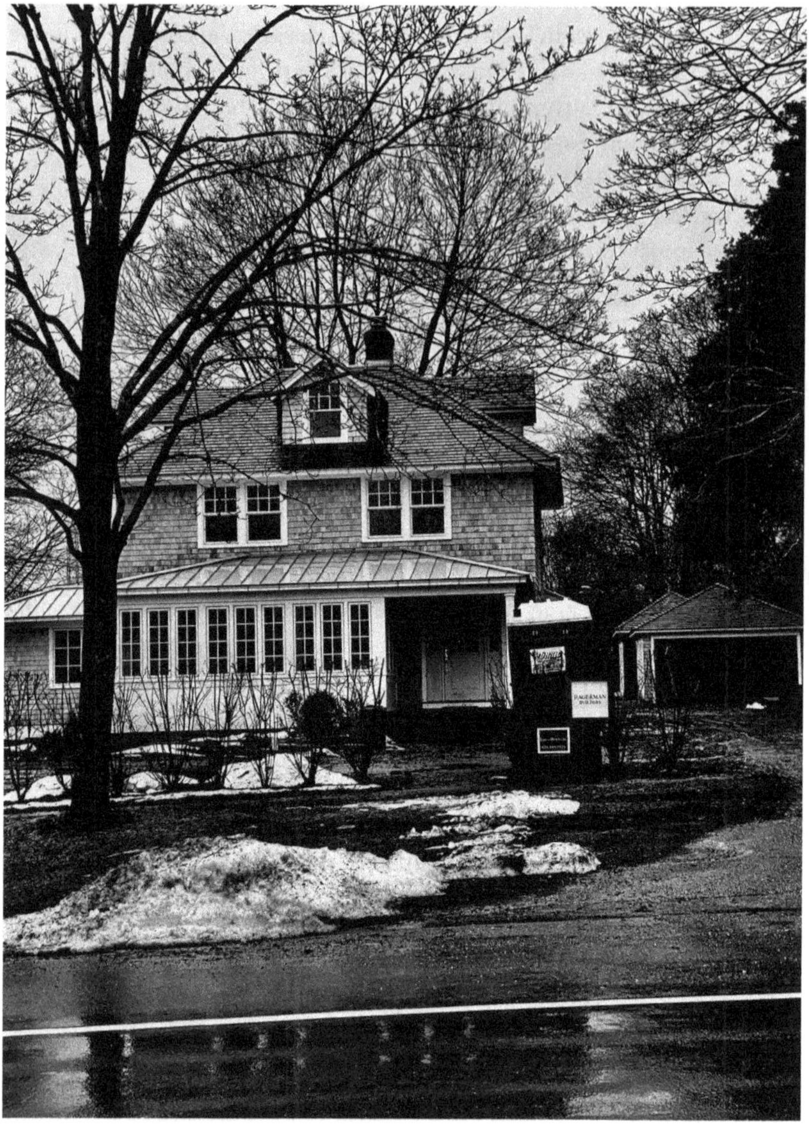

FIGURE 2 Pantigo Lane House, 1960

know that the rabbits came to live in the horse stable and made many more baby bunnies.[3]

We moved to our big house when Mom was pregnant with Randy, number six in the lineup. Before that our tiny house on Church Street had burst her seams, overflowing with children and dogs. Mom and Daddy Tom had one room, while my sisters Toni and Ann shared a room with me. Toni and I had bunk beds and Ann a crib. The third tiny room was shared by Tommy and Robin and their two cribs. I did love that house and its grounds, though both were tiny. I was little too, only six years old when we moved. Outside there was an apple tree which we loved to climb, and leafy overgrowth that was the perfect place for forts. When we arrived at the new house it was all set up, ready to go. We landed in this new land, another of Mom's amazing projects. The powder blue wall-to-wall carpet and the huge wrap-around couch with its light blue and white fabric was beautiful. However, it was not kid friendly. So, Mom put a plastic runner over the carpet that ran from the staircase to the kitchen. We were told to stay on its course. I think it would have been a good Mom idea to take a film of this first day, before the deluge of children. This room was almost immediately transformed.

## 3 The First Glimpse at My Princess Crown

I did not ask for the princess crown. I did not want to mother all your children. At thirteen years old, I wanted to be small, to be a child. No place for that for the eldest of seven. I wanted to be like them, not to lead them. I wanted to, at least, look like them; I wanted to belong. I wanted to be curious not cautious. I wanted to be watched out for, not to be always watching out. I hoped that someone might see me as a true child and mother me. My small frame helped me in the task of minimizing and presenting as a needy child.

There was a tiny children's clothing store, the Carousel Shop, in our town. I loved that store because it offered kid sized *Danskin* shorts and tops that I could fit into. *Danskin* was the desired label for outfitting the elementary school group. I had no interest in wearing teen clothes. I had no interest in the rites of passage available to me as a 13-year-old. Choosing to cross that threshold meant leaving behind the kingdom of the small. In that kingdom the small were cared for and loved. On the other side was the land of the caretakers. If only by adornment, I would resist the call to surrender.

I was in the tiny dressing room, in the tiny store, trying on tiny clothes that fit me just fine. I liked how young I looked in the mirror. Maybe I could pass for nine or ten. Who would expect a child of that age to do all the mothering? As I was leaving the dressing room, crossing the threshold, it happened. My body betrayed me. Passage. There it was. Without choice I was swept from the kingdom of the small on a carpet, that was not by my definition magic, into the realm of the unspeakable, into the realm of "women." There, in my tiny children's outfit, my period came.[4]

## 4 A Gift

Before the big house, there was our tiny house. Its surrounding neighborhood was filled with other small houses and many children. I do not remember much parental restriction. We were free to roam unattended. Around one of the bends lived an older girl, Olivia Habendorf. She was four years older than me, and compared to my age of six, she seemed like an adult. Olivia was beautiful and quiet, and I admired her. I wanted to take her home, to become her. I think I was hoping for a big sister, a guide, a mother. I admired her from afar and created stories about our shared life. Of course, I never told her about my feelings. This was my own story, one which could not be taken from me or altered in any way.

Somehow, during that time, a doll came into my possession. I am not sure if it was a gift to me, or something that was won in a game, or passed down from an older cousin. I think it was not passed down, because she was beautifully untouched and new, like my Olivia stories. She was a nun doll, complete with habit and cross. I am not or was Catholic, but somehow knew that Olivia was. Most Holy Trinity was around the corner from my house and my house sat on the walking path between Olivia's and mine. I watched her walk to church on Sunday mornings. I guessed that she must be Catholic. I was fascinated with her and with my doll's nun's habit: the black veil, with white head band, the long dress with the black socks and shoes that were revealed when I lifted the doll's skirt. She was a doll of many secrets. She was just like me although I was not Catholic. I loved her for the short time that she was mine.

If I could not speak to Olivia, at least I could give her this beautiful doll. But, if I were to offer it to her face to face, I would have to speak, to justify my offering. I needed another plan.

I decided that when she went off to church on Sunday, I would sneak around to her house and leave it on her porch. I was good at sneaking. On the third Sunday in July, off I went with my nun further swaddled in cloth. She looked now, like a baby Jesus nun doll. I wanted her to be protected and the wrapping was adornment that described her a package, as a gift, I thought. And it had to be clear that the doll was a gift for Olivia.

I never did find out what she thought about it. Like everything else in my Olivia stories, I got to make up the endings. So, in my story, Olivia found it, and searched the neighborhood for the giver. It was just like in Cinderella when the prince roamed the land with the glass slipper in search of its owner who would then be crowned princess. And like the prince, Olivia went from house to house with the doll, until she found me. Confronted, I acknowledged the truth. It was me. She decided to be my big sister and move in and take care of me. And then, we lived happily ever after.

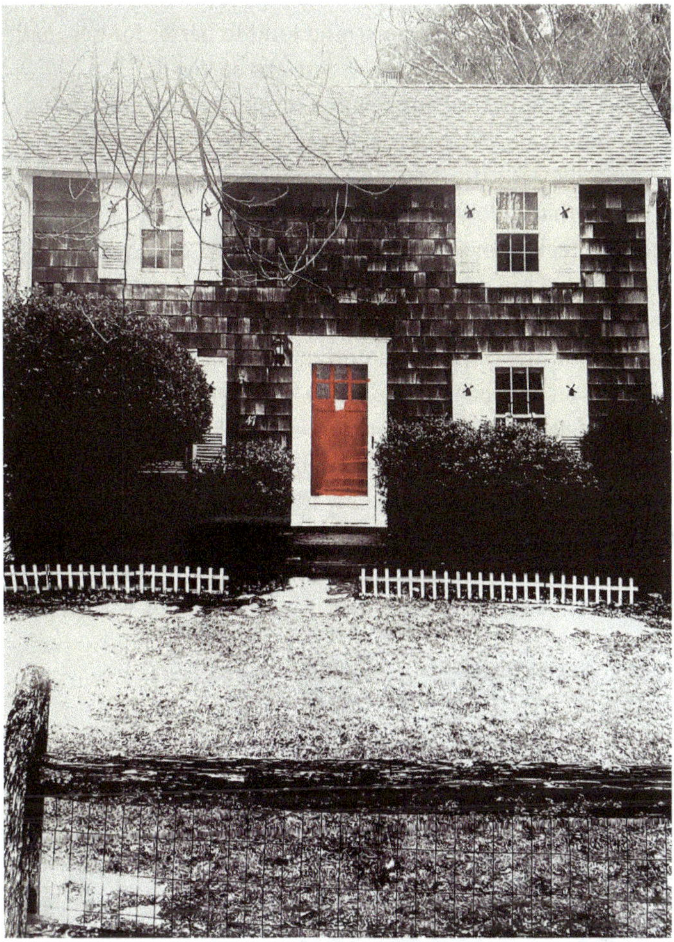

FIGURE 3 Church street house with red door, 1958

## 5 Mary Had a Little Lamb

She was always small. I can't remember exactly what she looked like as a puppy. Mitzi was a black poodle, and like my stories, she was mine. Unlike my stories, she was not a secret which meant she could be taken from me. She came to live with us shortly after we moved to the big house. She joined our sibling group of seven children, three dogs, two horses, one cat and many bunnies. Mitzi had long hair which meant she had to get haircuts, be daily brushed and routinely bathed. At first, we took her to the vet to be groomed but after a while my mother decided we should get dog clippers and trim her ourselves. *Ourselves* meant *me*. I must say her hairdos were quite unusual. I attempted to mimic poodle do's that I saw in books and on other dogs, but the results did not mirror their models. Mitzi didn't mind. Anything I did to her or for her made her happy. She didn't ask for much. She only wanted to be loved.

I rode my bike to school daily, to all my schools: primary, elementary, middle school, and high school. Every day Mitzi followed along. Every day Mitzi sat with my bike and waited for me to come out at the end of the school day. She was like the little lamb that followed Mary to school. Seeing her waiting for me every day made me feel so loved. She was always there, even when it was raining. I always thought of Mitzi when I heard that rhyme. Years later I used the tune for a dance I created for little children, with gestures of caring for baby birds. I had not thought of the connection until now. Love, tenderness, devotion, like braids, are woven between Mitzi and my little dance.

Her loyalty and her devotion were directed toward me, but she had plenty left to share. I remember that she lost a litter of pups because of some medical complication which left her unable to have any more. One day I found her in my closet. Tucked in close to her was a stuffed animal that she gently stroked and incessantly, almost desperately licked. I thought that she must have felt that it was her pup and she wanted to get it to nurse. Shortly after, we acquired

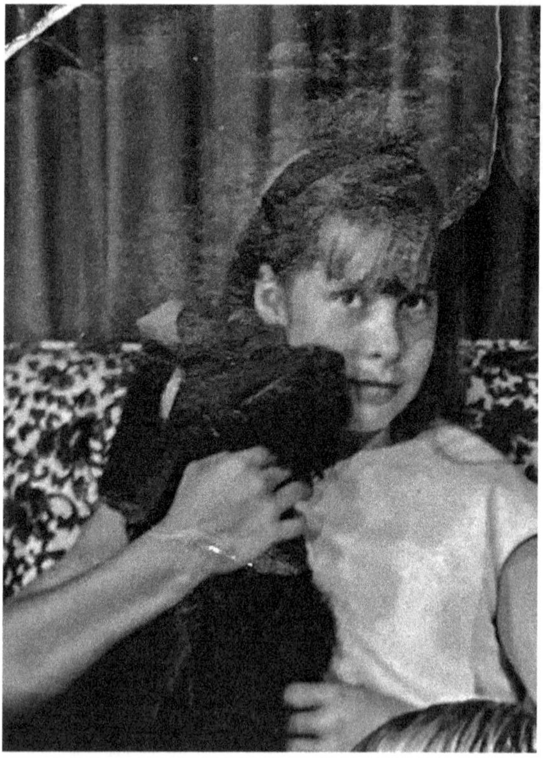

FIGURE 4 Mitzi and me, 1965

a kitten which Mitzi claimed as her own. She nursed that kitten until he grew to be her size. My mother also preferred babies to big children.

Leaving home for college meant leaving Mitzi behind. Leaving home meant someone else needed to attend to her long hair which left unattended, became a snarl of dreadlocks. This was before I knew what dread locks were, but in retrospect, they sure looked like dreadlocks. No longer a puppy, was she less appealing to my mother? Or was it that she required care if she was to look presentable? How she looked seemed important to my mother. When I came home for Spring break, Mitzi was gone. My loyal and precious friend, she that was mine, had been taken from me. Mother said that she had given her to friends who would love and care for her. My brother told me the truth: Mom had her put to sleep.

## 6 Best Friends

Maybe I should have kept my mouth shut. Or maybe I should have been less silly, more grown up. But I must say, Chelle Allendon was my best friend, and, with her, I thought, I could be my real self. Let down the princess crown, not pretend to be one of the Stroms, run crazy with her, like the ten-year-old child that I was. But to backtrack, my stepfather's last name was Strom and my real father's last name was Johnson. When my mother divorced, she moved us from Pennsylvania to East Hampton where she married my stepfather and had five children with him. When in certain company she told me to say that my last name was Strom. She didn't want those certain people to know that she had been married before. It was neater, more proper for me to slip in under the umbrella of her group of Strom children. Being a Johnson must be reserved for times spent with my father's family in Pennsylvania. So, back to Chelle. Hers was the perfect family. She had an older sister, Gay, and an older brother, Paul. Gay was beautiful and a cheerleader; Paul was the star quarterback on the high school football team. Her mother was the ideal mom. She was our Girl Scout troop leader. I loved being with her at her house. It was so peaceful. I can still picture every room in her house, especially Gay's. Gay was a goddess to me. Like Olivia, I looked up to her as the perfect grown-up girl. I don't remember ever having a conversation with her. I just watched her. She was the most popular girl in the high school. She was unapproachable for me, as I was just a clumsy little kid, a friend of her sister.

Word had it that Gay, now in college, was inviting Chelle and one of Chelle's friends, to come up and stay with her for the weekend. I could only imagine the bliss of a whole three days with my best friend and her goddess sister. I was the logical choice, at least in my mind. After all, I *was* the best friend.

Hanging out in Chelle's room, I tinkered about, looking at all her magical possessions. Her room was full of treasures. She had gone downstairs to talk with her mother about something. And then I found it. The letter from Gay. I hesitated but decided to read it. After all, it must have more information about our upcoming weekend. "I can't wait to see you and show you my school. It is heaven. We will have so much fun. Just one thing, please do not bring Dicki, anyone else would be fine." I felt, reading those words, as if my whole world had crashed in. I could not understand what was wrong with me, why Gay did not want me to come to her school. Was I an embarrassment to her? It felt like the embarrassment my mother felt acknowledging my true paternity. Over and over again I thought about potential shortcomings that I might have displayed. Too short, too loud, too big a family, not the right clothes. Nancy Babson was second in line for the role of Chelle's best friend. I think Gay chose Nancy. Years later, Nancy became captain of the cheerleaders. Whatever she had, I sure didn't. I am not sure, to this day, what that was.

Chelle and her mother made up some excuse for why I was to be excluded. Whatever the excuse was, it was constructed as an attempt to take away the sting of Gay's rejection. I know that it was not the true reason. I wish that I had been confident enough then to persuade them to tell me the truth. I can still feel the sting. It has left a tiny hole in my heart.

## 7 Sailing

We did not sail when I was growing up. Even though we lived on the ocean, we spent little time on it. Sailing was for the rich families who belonged to yacht clubs and wore white pants all thorough the summer. I don't think I ever had a pair of white pants until I got married and went to visit my father's clan in Pennsylvania for a post-wedding celebration, and thought that, as the bride I should wear a white pants suit.

So, I always told people who asked about my relationship to sailing, "I am a swimmer. I spent my time in the ocean not on it." Saying that made me feel like not sailing had been my choice. I created those choice stories for myself. Anyway, if I were to imagine or remember sailing, I picture myself, not on the water but above it, sailing through the sky. And I would not be alone because I really do not know how to sail. My sister Ann, now an angel, would be with me. I think that she did get to sail when we were kids because she was secretly dating Jimmy Poole, one of the rich summer boys who lived on Ocean Avenue in one of the mansions there. I remember her telling me a story about how she was invited to dinner there and did not know how to eat an artichoke. Sort of like the scene in "Pretty Woman" when the Julia Roberts character didn't know which pieces of silverware were meant for which food item.

Maybe it was because there were so many of us that Mom didn't teach us the etiquette that I know she was groomed with. I think that she sent me to her fancy boarding school, the one which all the women in her family for three generations attended, to learn table manners. Anyway, Ann never made it to that fancy school. She loved being home, and I imagine, she loved sailing. So, here she was at the helm, carrying us through the clouds. I am looking down and wondering what I have done, in my lifetime, of value. What I see right now has to do with sailing. Even though I married for love, not money, and ended up, for a while being a single mother, I did make sure that my children got to sail. What money I had was used to pay for good schools where they would meet people who knew how to sail. Off Nina went time and again, with Alexa's family, to Nantucket, to Nice. I don't know if she ever put it together that I had some part in making that happen. Later I came to live by the sea again, and there my son Dylan, *child of the waves*, learned to sail. He does well on the ocean as does Nina who surfs in California where sharks swim. They are both more courageous than I am.

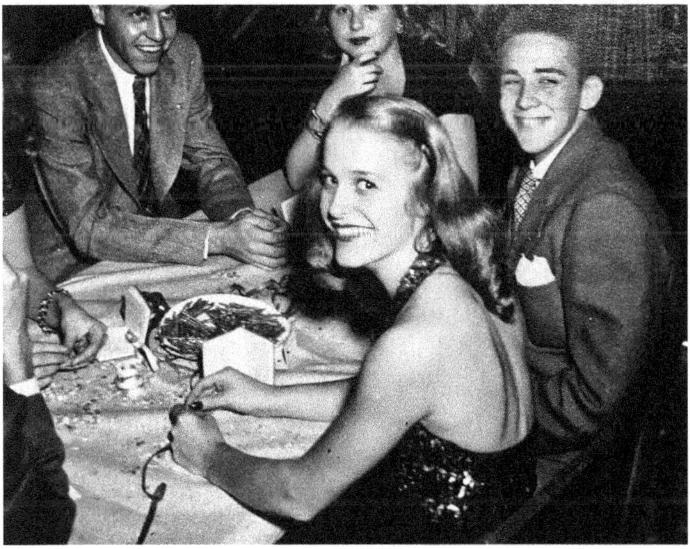

FIGURE 5 Mom at high school dance, 1946

## 8 Song

*The moment I wake up before I put on my makeup, I say a little prayer for you.* Burt Bacharach music was a constant, the audio background in our house of many. A child of the 60s, I drank the subliminal messages: a good girl was the girl who always looked pretty and was available, 24/7 for her man. Her life must be devoted to his pleasure. If she did not keep on her toes, he would look elsewhere. *Day after day there are girls at the office, and men will always be men....* I loved the sound of the music and didn't much take in the meaning of the words, but I knew them by heart. I can sing them all today. When I started to look like a woman, I know that I resisted surrendering to the look. I was horrified by voluptuousness. I wonder if my devotion to maintaining a childlike body was, in fact, a reaction to the script that I would be forced to assume, as a woman, as a wife. *Time to get ready for love.*

*All the leaves are brown, the leaves are brown, and the sky is grey....* Eighth grade dancing outside with Casey. Dusk promises the privacy of darkness coming. My nose is pressed against his tweed jacket, and I suck in the smell of English Leather. It is my new most favorite fragrance. Time has stopped. I'm not sure how I got here or if my parents know I am here. Other couples are dancing. Oh my god, I am part of a couple! Nothing matters except that he is holding me, and we are dancing to the most beautiful sound I have ever heard. The Mamas and Papas. I will never feel alone if they are singing.

*Oh yeah, I'll tell you somethin', I think you'll understand, When I say that somethin',I want to hold your hand, I want to hold your hand, I want to hold your hand.* Fourth grade. I am in Chelle's kitchen and her family is buzzing with excitement over this new musical group The Beatles. The big excitement seems to be their long shaggy hair. Chelle's older brother and sister are excited, her parents, not so much. The enthusiasm seems to spill over into every crack in every room of every place I move. In school my little vocal group, *The Cleff Dwellers*, decides to sing their big hit as a surprise in the choral concert upcoming. We have a secret... *Listen, do you want to know a secret, do you promise not to tell.* Our big secret is this: we, all six of us, Dicki, Chelle, Lulu, Barbara, Philip, and Lenny, decided that we would wear wigs that looked like the Beatles haircuts. We got mop tops and dyed them black. When it came time for the number, we whipped the wigs out from behind our backs and put them on. The shrills and screeches from the audience drowned out our singing. Years later our class, a very musical one, went on to win all the annual talent contests. Philip became a famous jazz musician who plays regularly at the Newport Jazz Festival. In between singing the Beatles and being a famous jazz musician, he played keyboards in my boyfriend David's rock group, *The Zoo. The Zoo* held weekly dances at the VFW and played the music of *The Doors, Cream, Crosby Stills and Nash, Jimmy Hendriks* and other 60s groups. As David was the lead singer, I had to dance with myself. The big excitement for me was the costume changes: I was a cheerleader and raced, in my cheerleading uniform to the VFW, and changed to cool dance clothes in the bathroom. I loved the drama of changing costumes.

## 9 Choir Love

Mother always sang in the choir. Singing is beautiful and romantic. In the movie *A Star is Born* (1976) Barbara Streisand and Kris Kristofferson face-to-face, sharing one mike, *sing* "Love soft as an easy chair, one love that is shared by two, I have found in you." Years later I hear the song played in the apartment below me, over and over, accompanied by the sobbing of the man whose lover has left him. Although I have felt the historic suppression of my metaphorical voice, I have always been a singer. I too, like all my sibs, sang in the choir. That, to me, was true community. Mom, who was one of the two soloists in the Presbyterian Church choir always sang "Oh Holy Night" at the candlelight service on Christmas Eve. That was the voice I hoped to inherit. So, I sang in the choir, took voice lessons weekly at my fancy boarding school as well as English riding lessons daily during fourth period, right before lunch. Mom was an accomplished equestrian. Her gifts placed her on a pedestal on which she stood, far removed from us, her children. We observed her in her respective lairs, but rarely entered them. I wonder what it was like for kids who had moms who sang with them rather than for them. Maybe that is why, as designated family princess servant, I began singing with my siblings. I started making plays with parts designated to them by me, with costuming and scenery all created by me.

## 10 Getting Hurt

The three steps that loomed before me should have been five. They seemed like a mountain. I am counting them and only find three. For my tiny body they appeared before me unsurmountable, worthy of a day's journey. A mountain of brick to climb with the reward at the top being my grandmother's house. My legs are too short, I think. I don't think that I can make it up these steps. Was it *bad manners* to say that I was afraid? I was only four years old, so I am not sure that I understand about *bad manners*. Somebody big, I think it was Uncle John, actually he was my step-uncle John standing beside me. But what was he doing there? Was this before my mother married Daddy Tom, my stepfather? I seem to remember that there was rumor that mom had dated them both before Ann was born. I am suspicious now, in retrospect. Was Uncle John Ann's father? Why was he there with us on that day?

Uncle John picks me up and put me on his shoulders. I am riding high. I am atop a camel. I am high to the sky. I am floating and can see so far. From my usual place on my own two feet, I can see less. Lots of legs and stomachs. Hands when hanging freely from arms. Walking hands and feet. I am floating in the lightness of my riding. Then a jolt. My face moves quickly closer to the bricks. Steps one two three. I am downed. Maybe he tripped or maybe he dropped me. The brick is hard and rough. My head is bleeding. A lot.

I am swept up in the arms of someone. Uncle John, I think. The medical center is close by, so we don't need to get in the car. It is a quick ride being carried in the man's arms. In his arms I am held down and can't see much.

Next all is bright and white. The doctor's office. I only see white and light. I know that stitches are put into my forehead cut. From where I am lying, I can see more that I did in the arms of the man. I look around and am wondering who else is there. Wondering and imagining keep me safe from what brought me there.

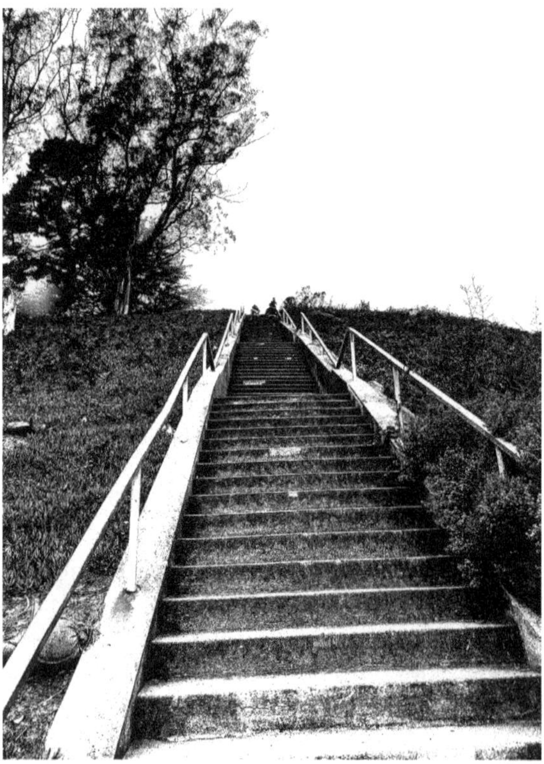

FIGURE 6 Too many steps

## 11 Fear

I am not afraid of cars. I love driving and the freedom that it provides. Freedom of responsibility. Freedom of thought. On wheels, like skateboards. Floating in between this and that, both states requiring me to be present. While driving I can be anywhere in time. I can drift backwards where I reclaim old loves, human, architectural, geographical. I can jump forward, but usually, only for a moment. The freedom of driving means that I don't, while in transit, have to plan anything. Liminal. Crepuscular.

But I do find cars popping up when I remember fear. Unraveling time, like a surprise ball, I am first in a tiny, borrowed Honda. It is 1982 and I am driving with my husband Paul down the coast of California. A vacation. We have left baby Nina with my sister in Mendocino and are headed for LA. We are driving highway 101, which is claimed to be one of the most beautiful in America. It serpentines along the rocky coast and provides vistas, at some points, a mile down to the ocean. Paul is driving, so I am sitting in the passenger seat. The road is narrow and the drop down to the ocean is deep. I think I have always been afraid of heights especially if there is no barrier between me and the depth. Falling, crashing, dying? I am not sure which fear predominates but I am not able to breath. I am having a panic attack. My feet are braced on the roof of the car. We stop and I get out, just to have my feet on the ground for a moment. Loss of control. Like on a roller coaster. I have never been able to ride them. Or a Ferris wheel. I see myself sitting in one of the little cars. I am stuck at the top and someone begins to rock the car. The feeling is similar to my highway 101 ride. I need to get out and stand on the ground. Grounded I am calm.

The image of fear housed in a car carries me back to a drive to Pennsylvania. I am four years old. Maybe five because there are at least three children in the car besides me. It is very dark and cold. I think it must be Thanksgiving or Christmas and we are *en route* to my maternal grandparent's home in Pennsylvania. The road serpentines continually upward. We are in the mountains and somehow, I know that we have snow chains on our tires.

Then again, it must be before snow tires were invented. I remember the sound of the chains as the tires turned. My mother and stepfather were discussing the chains. We children were all in the back of the car with the seats folded down. The back of the car seemed really big and was full of blankets for our makeshift and communal bed. Mom was insistent upon an annual trip to her parents' home. There she showed us off and had a portrait taken of us all for our Christmas card. So, it must have been Thanksgiving that the trip was made. What made me afraid was the snowstorm that we moved through. The sound of the chains, the slow rate at which Daddy drove, the whispers my parents shared, the darkness. Mom told us not to move so much. Looking out the window I saw many pine trees framing the road. The deep again. I see down below which is very far.

I don't think I was old enough to know what it meant to be out of control. Somehow the sounds of the chains and my parents' whispers were new sounds. Familiar sounds are safe sounds, and I could not hear any of them on this car ride.

## 12 The Chauffeur

Before the trip through the mountains in the car, there was a time that we moved to my grandparents' home in Pennsylvania. I was in kindergarten, so I must have been about five years old. My only siblings that joined me would have been Toni and Ann who were four and one. The others had not been born yet. I don't see any moving pictures of the three of us. I only see me. I had been taken out of kindergarten and was finishing my school year in a kindergarten there. My teacher at home had my classmates send me letters with pictures attached. I really missed being home. I was told that we moved there so Daddy could go to business school and so he and I could get our tonsils out together. I don't know if the two events were connected but those are the two events that left me with pictures and stories.

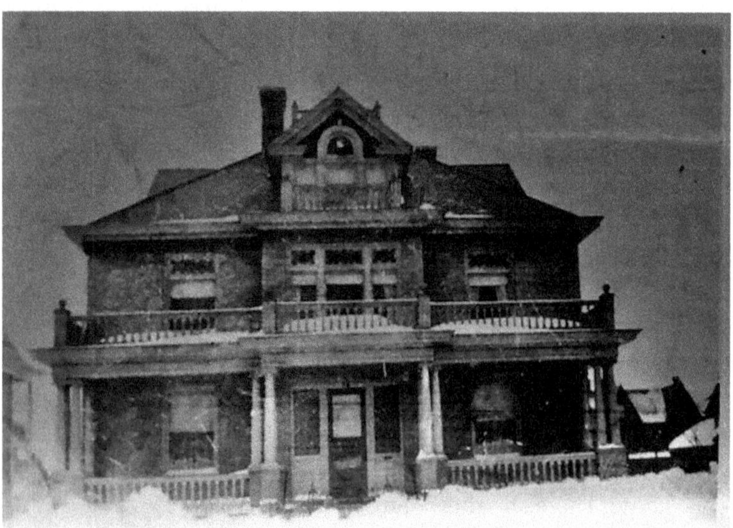

FIGURE 7 Bom Bom's house

My grandparents lived in a big house that had three floors and an elevator. I know they were rich, but I don't remember being with them, only watching them. They were very old. My mother was the youngest of ten children. Her older siblings had children that were her age. There was a beautiful grape arbor in the backyard and the housekeeper would take me outside to play under it. I do remember her and her kindness toward me. The other person that became my buddy was Dominick the chauffeur. He drove me to kindergarten every day and picked me up when school was over. Did I make friends there? I don't see them in this story. Maybe it was because of the limo they saw me arrive in. I know that this was pretend life, not my real one.

My Daddy Tom and I went to the hospital together to get our tonsils out. Despite the nice nurses and ice cream, I knew I needed to escape. I am not sure where I thought I was going but knew what I was leaving. I crept out of my room one night and made it as far as the elevator. Early entrapment. This may be the first time I felt like I was in prison, I was living someone else's pretend life and was someplace that did not feel like home. That I don't remember my mother or my sister being there makes me think that I maybe I was dreaming. Sometimes I was confused about real life and dream life.[5]

## 13 Corn

I do know that some moms spent a lot of time in the kitchen making food. My mom was not one of those moms. I don't remember cookbooks at our house. Mom liked to make holiday meals. And her recipes were in her head. She did not follow cooking rules. She made us the special meals that she said were passed down in her family. Corn pudding, her mother's recipe, was a Thanksgiving and Christmas staple. We watched her, all standing in the kitchen, as she recited out loud, what went into making our corn pudding. Somehow it seemed that it gave her a connection to her dead family. I remember my grandparents as cold and distant. Later when we grew up, we would call Mom on Thanksgiving and Christmas from our respective homes so that she could recite the recipe steps to us. We never wrote the recipe down. I think it was one of the few rituals that she shared with us, so we cherished them.

I lost my first tooth biting into an ear of corn. Before my father's fields became pastures for horses, they were for corn. The little farm in Pennsylvania that he bought had a silo. It is no longer there. It was filled with corn to feed the animals. I wonder what animals lived there. I was six when he moved from the little city to the country. It was a place for me filled with mystery. I spent half of every summer at his farm with his new family, my other three half siblings.

It was so different from my mother's home by the sea. I loved running through the cornfields and stopping to husk an ear and take a bite. We were not supposed to do that. There was a magic for me finding a hidden place in the fields where no one could see me. There I could sit an imagine anything, and eat the forbidden fruit, an ear of uncooked corn. It was a fully cooked and grilled ear that took my first tooth. And I was not alone but in the company of a large group. Maybe it was Daddy's birthday. There was always a big party for him. He was born on the Fourth of July.

Maize is a staple food in many cultures other than mine. Native American, Mexican, I believe. It is made from corn. It seems that corn had grown wild on its own in our American fields before someone decided that there was a better more profitable use for those fields. I think that corn is full of truth. What is true sustains us, without fanfare or fancy additives. No recipes, just simple honest truth.

As an offering to the starving children in Bangladesh, years later, my school donated to the cause all the money spent to feed students for a day. I had been sent away to boarding school. It was part of our legacy, my mother's legacy, to attend this school. Her mother, her sisters, her aunts, my female cousins all attended. I was chosen, as the oldest daughter to follow in their footsteps. I felt like the sacrificial lamb. It was not my choice. I remember that mom told me that the cooks there were Amish and that they all used very rich recipes. Shoofly Pie was one of those recipes. Mom told me that for sure I would get fat eating their food. I don't know why she told me that. I decided that I would not get fat, so from day one, I ate almost nothing. On that day, the day of offering to the starving children in Bangladesh, we were ordered to eat cornmeal mush instead of our regular three meals. To the other students, eating corn meal mush and sacrificing three hearty meals was experienced as denial. To me who had eaten nothing for months it was a feast. I remember still how incredible the warmed and soft corn tasted, how it nourished my starved and empty body. I still remember the taste and the smell of that warmed corn. I thought about the waste in our country and how the excessive amassing of possessions made it impossible to appreciate any gift. Self-denial for me became a distorted prerequisite for being worthy of a nourishment of any kind. But on that day, I had no choice but to eat. And it was corn, the gift of truth.

## 14 My Dream Play

*The Sound of Music*. The story, the characters, these were the places and people of my dream. Seven Children. We had all the characters. Could I still be Maria? Her dance with the Captain wherein their shared glance of acknowledgement, told us of love. And then there was the dream wedding with all the nuns looking on and singing the processional. As the oldest child I took it upon myself to stage the play. Like my stories, I was in control of the outcome and the part which I would play in it. For three or four years I planned for the summer production of *The Sound of Music*. At my grandmother's summer home in Eagles Mere, Pennsylvania I share time with siblings and many young cousins. They would become my actors. Each winter I made the costumes. I had learned to sew in home economics class and was pretty good at making things without patterns. Each winter I cast the characters, with me, of course, as Maria. In my plays, I could always cast myself as the heroine. My sister Toni, who was a year younger than me, but a bit bigger, would always be the Captain. We could practice over the winter and spring and be ready to teach the little ones their songs and parts.

My grandmother's house was a big Queen Anne-style house with a wraparound porch. It was the perfect setting for our play. 1965. All that we needed was an audience. My grandmother, who had been an actress, was proud of her grandchildren and their shared production. She invited all of her Ladies Club members to attend our show. What made me feel most successful about this event was the fact that my daddy decided he would have our program printed at his office. This offering made me feel as if he was proud of me. I often felt that his new family was the source of his pride. When he was angry at me, he told me that I was "just like my mother." But here, as I produced the play, directed it, costumed it and presented it to his mother's friends, I was perfect in his eyes.

Every winter following the first production, my siblings and cousins expressed excitement for the next year's production. Of course, every year we did *The Sound of Music*. Of course, every year I was Maria.

## 15 Storms

Today it was cold and windy. It made me think of storms past. Childhood storms. Communion. Those storms that brought us together. I don't much remember times spent with my brothers and sisters. Flashes of shared pranks. My mother was a trickster and loved to play jokes on neighbors and friends. She passed on that gift. We are all now trickers. That is something we share, that sense of humor. Ours has a dryness to it that we recognize immediately in others. If they shared our form of humor, they become our kin.

As for storms, they housed the backdrop for intimacy and engagement. Hurricanes were frequent and recurrent in our ocean town. We did not fear them as they were expected and seasonal. Like snowstorms. When we knew they were coming we prepared by walking to the beach as an army (there were seven of us). Watching the ocean transform from its usual welcoming and beckoning surf to one which sang a violent warning "keep out." From the safe distance that the dunes provided, we watched and listened. We knew that in Montauk at the end of our island, which was surrounded on two sides by sea, that storm watching was not safe. Residents had to evacuate and climb to the high point of the town. Montauk Manor sat upon what we considered to be a mountain. The exodus. Lowlanders found respite on that mountain.

When the storm was finding its eye, we would go home. Watching small trees and shrubbery fly by, out of windows like televisions, we shared the entertainment. But, best of all, the electricity usually went out. We hoped for that each time we shared a hurricane. This meant that we all had to sleep downstairs in the living room in front of the fireplace. The fire light made magical the shared time. We told scary stories, jokes and food that could be cooked over the fire. Without electricity we found no distraction from each other. On regular days each of us took our separate paths away from the fire that had now burned out.

Storms of our childhood were safe storms. Grown now, I am finding that our storms are no longer predictable. We are no longer safe in our shelters. Maybe that is why we no longer share the pleasure of participating in the transformations that storms bring.

## 16 Gold Lame

There are many kinds of princess crowns. Some bring with them afflictions; others are symbolic objects for anointing or initiating some positive transformation. Adornment differs as interpreted by she that is adorned and by they that are her witnesses. Cinderella was a princess who wore her crown first as an affliction. In silence she, oppressed by greed and jealousy, was forced into servitude and into the wearing of rags. Her true crown was as invisible as was her silenced voice.

Half of my childhood was spent in the oasis mountain town Eagles Mere. Nestled, literally, at the pinnacle of a mountain, the nest of a town wrapped around a pristine lake. Here Marmie, my daddy's mother, maintained a Queen Anne summer mansion that was vacation home to all her progeny and to their children. Arriving, I left my Cinderella crown at my mother's home. Here I was free to roam through the pink parlor window seats that Marmie filled with amazing costumes. Daddy told me that Marmie was an actress before she was a mom and she brought all her costumes with her, maybe to remind her of wearing them on stage.

*Gold lame',* even as a five-year-old, I knew her name. There she rested, waiting for me to find her, deep inside the window seat with all her gorgeous friends.

Marmie told us that they were from Broadway. Auntie Kirwin, her sister, was a hat designer for Hollywood actresses. Some of her little wonders found a new home in the pink window seats. There were many choices for adornment. The princess I chose to be on that day was the princess, Eliza Doolittle. She shared with Cinderella the two-faced crown of dark and light.

The gold lame swirled out, in my hand like a bolt of lightning. I wrapped myself into its luminous sparkle and danced out of the room into the bright light of the green hillock outside. "I could have danced all night." As I sang the song, I felt myself transforming. There was magic inside of me. I needed no magic wand. My wand was invisible, and I believed in it. I was so happy letting the magic come out of me. And then the clock struck twelve. Crashing into the beautiful light came a dark and thunderous voice: "What are you doing? You are not supposed to be here. Everyone is down the hill celebrating my birthday. That is where you are meant to be. Get out of that outfit." Back to the rags. My father had not seen the magical me that was shining with the help of the gold lame. He only saw that I was not following the rules.

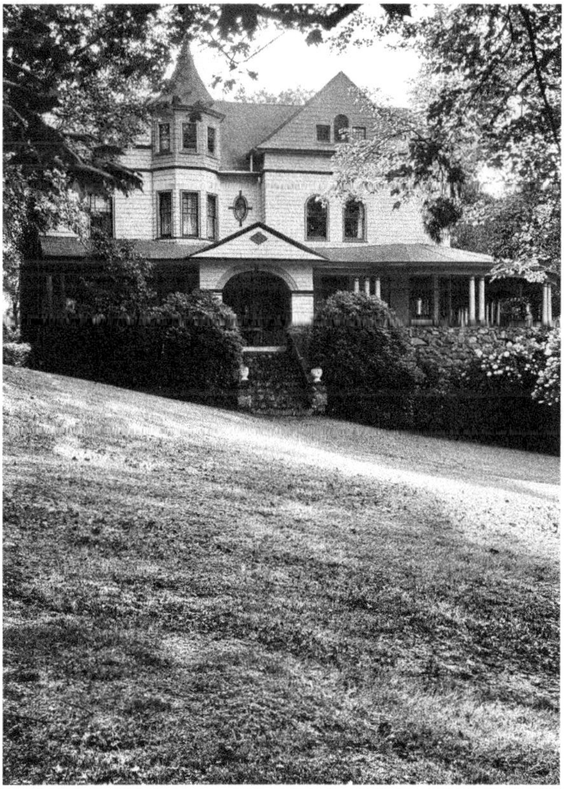

FIGURE 8 Marmie's house

## 17 Blue Baby

My exodus from dark to light was forced. I was not ready to leave the warmth of my mother's womb, my safe place for those nine months. Do I remember floating wrapped around myself in that translucent bubble? Did the muffled sounds of the world of light offer welcome? I imagine that time was like my grownup wakeful dreaming. That liminal state between the dark of night and the abrupt awakening that mornings force upon me, reminds me of my birth. I do not like leaving my bed. I did not like leaving my warm place inside of my mom's belly. I am most happy returning to my bed at night. Did I want to return to Mom's body? Did the light come too soon?

I was born blue. There was an actual term for babies born in the 50's and 60's that were not moving out on their own: *Blue Babies*. Medical intervention was the default during that time. Efficiency of time and sterility of place were advancements of modern-day science and birthing. The dialog of shared journey for mother and her fetus were forsaken. My mother always told us how difficult her pregnancies and labors were. She talked about having us kids as if she was a martyr. She became a saint in our eyes, and sometimes we felt guilty for making her go through so much to bring us into the world. For sure I was terrified to give birth, assured that I would follow her genetic path.

As children we believed that our parents could do no wrong and would tell no lies. I was an innocent. I believed in what I understood to be my mother's truths. I was a blue baby, and I was not ready to join her world. Dark has become symbolic of all things evil. Light on the other side, good. So, of course, it was desired that we move away from the dark toward the light. Babies were not allowed to stay too long in that dark place. The hidden. All things hidden are equated with femaleness. The doctors, most likely male doctors, determined when the time was right for babies to leave their dark homes and enter their world of polished light.

I was not ready, and no one was listening to me.[6] My mother too was brainwashed by the doctors. They were most likely handsome, and she must have let them know how much she was suffering in the pregnancy. So, they pulled me out and I was not ready to breath. I made no sound. I had no voice. The sound of my singing was left inside my dark and warm home. I know that this story, told to me by my mother, with most probable embellishment, held some element of truth. I still have the mark of forced removal between my eyes: *Forceps Marks*. I imagine the act of pulling a resistant animal toward danger or death. The animal knows what to avoid. My mother often pointed out my mark to her friends. Her labors were more difficult than anyone's and my mark made her story real. The mark has faded from its purplish red to light pink. It flares to its original darkness when I cry.

**Attunement**

Syncopation,
Ta-da-ta-da-ta-da-da-da
Within my dark and watery home,
I knew no chaos, no storm,
Only your heart sound,
Its syncopation,
Ta-da-ta-da-ta-da-da-da.

Seasick,
Taaaaaaaaaaaaaaa-da
Are those pulled too soon,
From the womb.
Lost was your heart sound,
Seasick I am
Without-taaaaa-it.

Syncopation,
Ta-da-da and Ta-da
Music all around sings
The heart songs lost.
The dance of the wave
My momentary medication.
Ta-da-ta-da-ta-da-da-da

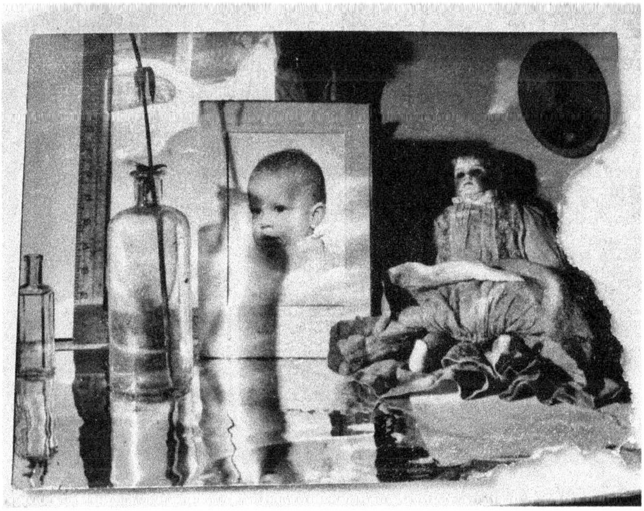

FIGURE 9 My mirrors, 1970

## 18 The Heart of the House

She was not positioned, like a river, to carry the everyday flow of running children and dogs. She was set back between the dining room and the main entrance way. Like a heart, she was a chamber with two openings, one for entrance and one for exit. Mostly, the flow was around her, not through her. Like a woman she transformed with the need affixed to her. She was not adorned in any permanent manner. She had no furniture that defined her as a functional room. Yet, she was a heart and so, from her emanated a steady pulse and song.

I see the hi-fi console with mom's record collection stacked upon it. The hi-fi was always alive with songs, especially those written by Burt Bacharach. I know all the words to most of the songs because they were played over and over. Here are a few lines from one of them:

> Day after day
> There are girls at the office
> And men will always be men
> Don't send him off with your hair still in curlers
> You may not see him again
> For wives should always be lovers too
> Run to his arms the moment he comes home to you
> He's almost here
> Hey! Little girl
> Time to get ready for love.

I spend a lot of time in the room, looking at the album covers, listening to the songs, singing them, dancing to them, imagining myself dressed like my mother. I picture her years before at her dressing table. I am three years old, and she is dressing for a date. She is beautiful and becomes more so as she combs her hair and fixes her makeup. The woman on the album covers looks like her. For example, Sharon Tate was a pregnant beauty that was killed in a horrific massacre by Charles Manson. There was hate and confusion about beauty during that time. My mother looked rather like Sharon. I did not understand why men sang about how women should look, and act then became angry at them when they followed the rules. All of the songs that pealed from that room rang the same gospel: be pretty, care for your man, make nice food, smile and don't argue. I wonder if my mother played those lyrics to convince herself, to keep herself at rein, or to find respite from the role of mothering seven children. *While combing my hair now, and wondering what dress to wear now, I say a little prayer for you. Together, together, that's how it must be. To live without you would only mean heartbreak for me.*

The little heart room was also a birthing chamber. Mom surrounded herself with pets. Her Irish Setter, Chula, was pregnant so she had a big box made that fit snuggly inside the room. Her birthing box. On the day that Chula was ready to deliver, mom had just returned from the hospital having had her gall bladder removed. She had a lot of unusual illnesses some of which were real. She was wearing an amazing black velvet long robe, I remember. She always wore beautiful clothes even when she was sick. I was in middle school at the time that I was called to the office. "You need to go home and deliver the puppies." My younger brother Tommy got the same call.

Chula was not an intuitive mother. As each puppy was entering the world, with the assistance of Tommy and me, unlikely midwives, and the chosen Princess and prince, or maybe the knaves or drone bees to mother's Queen, Chula would stand up and try to leave the box. She was not convinced by Burt Bacharach. She wanted her freedom. What was she to do with twelve puppies? Mitzi, my dog, as you remember, lost a litter of puppies, and could have no more. She jumped in the box, wrapped herself around the needy babies, and let them nurse on her. No milk, but lots of warmth and intention. The room housed the needy and the willing. The beautiful ones ran just when what was needed could only be fulfilled by them. I was thinking that Chula was just like Mom. Both were beautiful and good at birthing babies but not so good at staying to taking care of them. Chula showed us her escape plan. She bolted out of the box as soon as the puppies came out of her. Mom's escape was more of a secret. She made it look like she wanted to take care of the kids, but I think she wanted to run like Chula.

## 19 Barbara the Rebel

Barbara, my mother's best friend, came roaring into town on a motorcycle. I see a scarf trailing, like the tail of a kite. Her arms are wrapped around the driver who sits in front of her. The whole town appears to be watching her return to town. She had moved to New York City, gotten divorced, and then remarried a handsome younger troubadour. This sequence of events proved to be scandalous for our small town in the 1960's. I was seven or eight at the time and only knew that I was captivated by this figure.

At home we knew that it was important to be pretty and compliant. All of the songs which mom played at home told us so, but Barbara had left town and the proper marriage to marry a wild guitar player who had no money. Was

I captivated by the gossip or by the image of her zooming into town on the motorcycle? We didn't see many motorcycles on Main Street in East Hampton. I think once a group of greasy looking guys sped through on motorcycles headed for Montauk. You expected them to be riding those motorcycles, not a beautiful young woman.

Rules were being broken by Barbara. How much of this could I have understood as a girl of seven? I just remember being swept away by her at that moment. Somehow, I understood rebellion. Hers was not veiled, muffled, disguised. She wore her scarlet letter proudly and made no excuses. She had no reason to pretend. She was above all of that. And her assertiveness and confidence are what I admired, what I wanted for myself. But not for now. I was a rule follower. Only in my stories of make-believe did I imagine myself to be that bold and brazen heroine. I would put this plan away for later. Maybe their relationship allowed for the rebellion which mom was forced to hide at home.

Barbara's mother was a well-known soprano who sang with the Metropolitan Opera. Barbara spoke as if she too was an opera singer, with slow precision and perfect grammar. Barbara, like mom, sang in the choir, but they sang in different choirs. Our church was the Presbyterian one, Barbara was Episcopal. I always thought that Barbara's church was the more magnificent of the two. It was made of fabulous stone while ours was white painted wood. It seemed that there was more excitement in the stone church; the rituals were racier, the adornment and costuming more flamboyant. I think that dramatic plays were sometimes held in her church. The Presbyterians were more conservative. The events held within, predictable.

Everything that Barbara was involved in seemed to enhance the rebel I imagined her to be. She was an Aquarius like my mother. On paper they looked to be twins. However, Mom's mirror image was clandestine rather than revealed. She might have been equally rebellious but would never admit it. Lies are understood by children even if the understanding is unconscious. I wanted to be like Barbara. I watched her, maybe with the hope that I might assume some of her traits later. For now, I could only watch. I loved watching her perform for our local theatre events. She sang this song:

> I'm a poor little lamb who's lost in the woods, I know I could, always be good with someone to watch over me. Although he may not be the man some girls think of as handsome, to my heart he carries the key... so hurry and put on some speed, oh how I need, someone to watch over me.

She knew how to play the part, she could sing the song with lyrics acceptable, but I knew she didn't fall for them, not for one minute. She could break the rules if she sang the proper tune for her audience. She was the master, not the mistress.

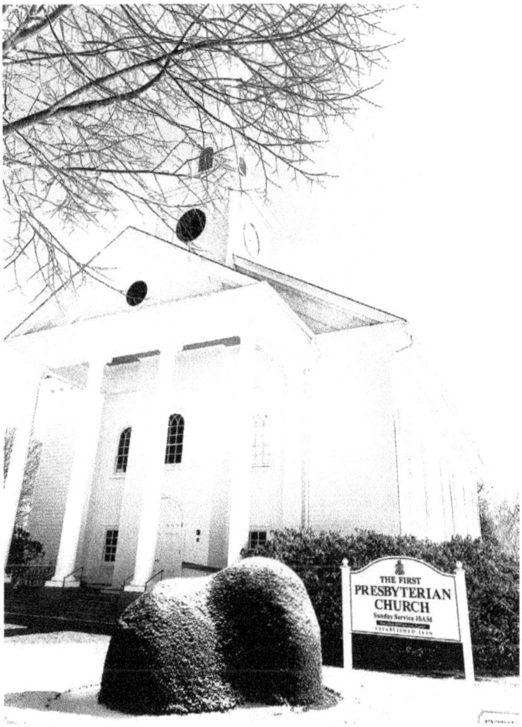


FIGURE 10
Mom's Presbyterian Church

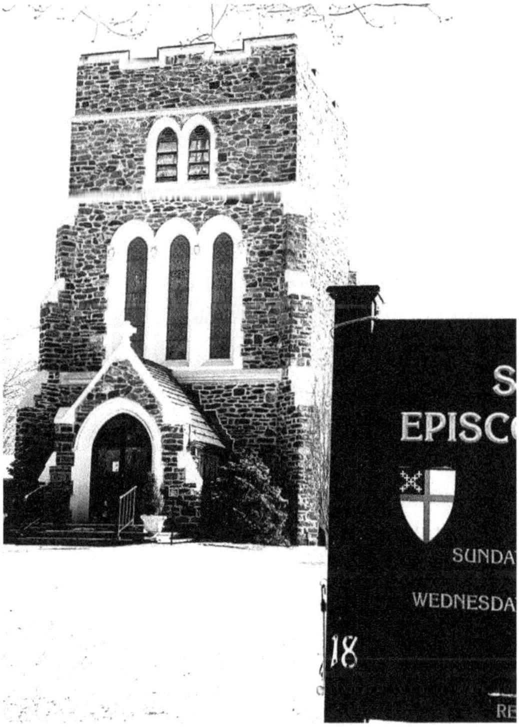


FIGURE 11
Barbara's Episcopal Church

## 20 The Prom Gown

Our Pantigo House was so big that it felt like a castle to me. The top floor was a world unto itself. Although the top floor had three bedrooms and a working bathroom, it was used only for storage. Seven children created the need for lots of storage. Mom got rid of most everything we no longer used. Clothes were the exception. She kept them all, hers and ours. One of the rooms was my playground. It housed the indoor version of outside raked leaves piled high. Like the haystacks at Daddy's farm, they were made just for us, for jumping on and into. Mountains of clothes provided us with a place to climb, caves to dig into, and when fallen and scattered, challenged us to rebuild, remembering how the mountain had been constructed.

We were not supposed to go up to the third floor. Somehow, disrupting the order was frowned upon. Maybe Mom was afraid we would smother in those mountains. Maybe the past was meant to be put way, to be unseen, to be forgotten but not destroyed. Why did she keep all those clothes if we were not going to wear them and could not play in them?

I was fascinated with what was hung rather than scattered. All of mom's clothes from her debutant days were collected and placed in plastic bags. They adorned the mountains of clothes like icicles on winter walls. Inside these icicles were beaded gowns, silk capes and velvet skirts which were truly the adornments of royalty. No one I knew wore such things. I loved taking them out, one at a time, holding them, and sometimes, putting one on. There were stories I could act out in these gowns. I imagined being at her school where everyone dressed like her, not just for dress up, but for everyday life. She told us, with pride, how everyone called her "Jinx" because she was a jinx to boys. She claimed to have been going steady with five at a time with each thinking that they were "the only." Of course, she was blond and beautiful.

There was one gown that looked like one of my Barbie doll's dresses. It was described on the box as her "prom gown." It was white, satin, strapless and fitted completely to the ankles where it flared out like a beautiful fan around her feet. A big red rose rested at the threshold of fabric which folded into the fan. If another color, or diaphanous, it would have resembled a mermaid dress. It was my favorite. Years later when I got sent off to the fancy girls' boarding school that mom, her sisters, her aunts, her mother and her great aunts had all attended, I asked mom to include in my wardrobe, a prom gown. As I was the chosen daughter to carry on the matriarchal legacy, she wanted me to dress just right. So, we got me the prom gown. It was not a duplicate of hers but was very close. Mine was shaped like hers but was made of white lace rather than satin. Lace was more popular than satin in the 1960's. I never did wear my prom gown because I left the school for home before prom time in the spring.

Years later, Mom's satin jewel of a gown was the only thing, other than all my parents' liquor, that our house cleaner, Lucy Mae Palmer took when she left the state of New York and her job with our family.

## 21 Mom's Dressing Table

The staircase is so very tall. It is inside of a tower. It is steep, narrow and high: Sleeping Beauty might be in a small room, hidden at the top of such a staircase. She is sitting at her loom. She looks at her work. She does not notice me. I am looking up from the bottom. There are so many stairs and I have such small legs. I am two and a half years old. At the top of my staircase is another small room. It is behind a light green carved door. The door opens. I am not opening it as I am still looking up from the bottom of the stairs. Does the wind creep behind to open it or is someone else in the room at the top? I only see my mother. She is sitting at a dressing table, looking in her mirror. She does not notice me. I am very quiet.

Mom is putting on her makeup. She is getting dressed to go out on a date. I watch her as she carefully paints her face. She is wearing curlers and beautiful under garments. I sense her excitement even though I am too young to understand what going out on a date entails. I do know that she is very pretty, with blond hair and blue eyes. I came into the world with my father's brown hair and green eyes. My younger sister Toni has mom's coloring. Toni is just one year old.

We have just moved away from our home in Pennsylvania. We have left my father behind and are in a new place that looks and feels very different. Here the world is flat and there is an ocean close by; in Pennsylvania there were mountains and rivers. Someone told me that we are here because my grandparents had vacationed here, and Mom wanted to move someplace "far away." She is beginning her new life and has taken us along. I imagine that in this new life she will have lots of dates. My teenaged cousin *Big Randy* is living with us for the summer as he has a job at Main Beach being a lifeguard. Maybe he is our babysitter while mom goes out on her dates. Later that summer, Randy broke his arm in the ocean rescuing someone doing his lifeguard job. I am not sure how he continued to be our babysitter. I don't see anything else from this time. I don't see us being with Mom, only her getting ready at that dressing table and mirror to go out. At two and a half, I am only watching others as if they are characters onstage in a play and I am sitting down in the audience.

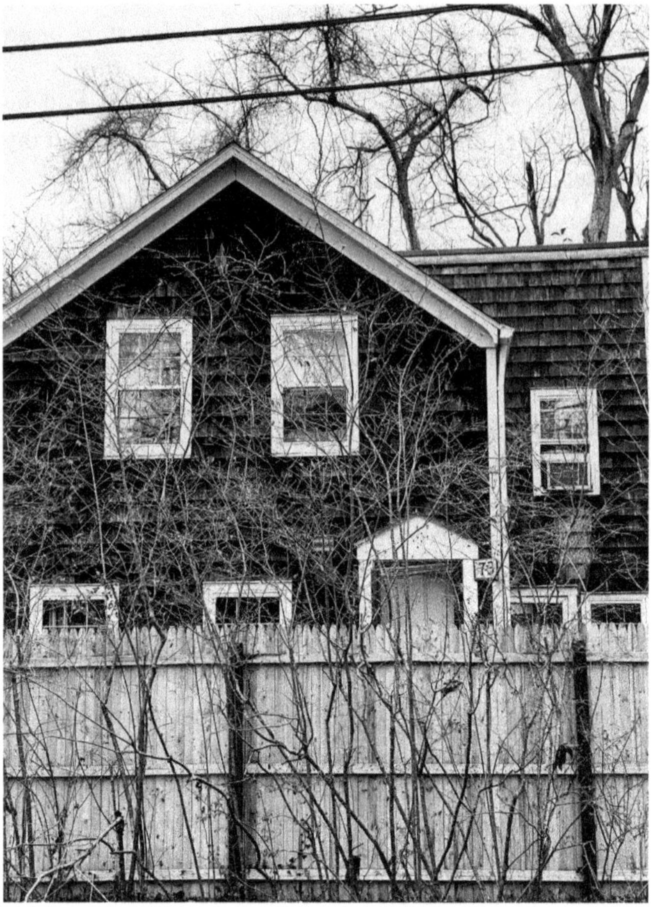

FIGURE 12 Mom's dressing room window, 1954

## 22 The Helpers Club

When I was in fourth grade, my cousin Barb and I decided we wanted to be Candy Stripers at the local hospital. I think, for me, it was all about the costume: pink and white striped dress with a white pinafore over it. I really wanted to have that costume. So, we formed this club that would somehow, in our minds, assure our acceptance into the coveted realm of Candy Strippers. I think we were too young to be accepted, but we were determined to be on the path toward that fame. Another part of being in the Helpers Club is that we were going to raise money to buy toys for the children in the hospital. I am not sure how we raised money but somehow, we did and somehow, we took toys to the hospital.

We decided to meet in Uncle Jacky's office to work on our helping projects. I think we were considering other ways we might help the community. Maybe collecting food for poor people. I am not sure if Barb was motivated to meet in her father's office because it would make us feel like we were doing some real work of value if we met in a real office, or if there was another motive for choosing this meeting place.

Once behind closed doors we were privy to the contents of Uncle Jacky's desk drawer: Playboy Magazines. Uncle Jacky, of all my uncles, was the most devout Christian. So, finding these magazines that had pictures of sexy naked women was a surprise. I could not figure out then why he would be hiding these magazines and looking at them when no one could see him doing so.[7] I was coming to understand that many grownups had secret lives that remained hidden and not discussed. For us, the world of those secrets was a new and exciting playground. We started to meet more than weekly for the Helpers Club whose members were learning about what grownup sexy women looked like and what grownup men wanted their women to do. In secret. Aunt Jane did not look like those Playboy Bunnies. She wore an apron and cooked amazing meals. We all liked going to their house for dinner because of her meals and her kindness. Mom was not such a good cook, or maybe she was, but didn't cook much. My stepfather Tom, Uncle Jacky's brother, was the cook in my new family. He made meals that mom didn't like and which she criticized in front of us all. Spicy spaghetti sauce, sausages, grits, are a few meals that I remember her criticizing. We loved his food. Anyway, I am not sure what mom was doing during the time she could have been preparing dinner. And I am not sure what Aunt Jane would have thought about the magazines in Uncle Jacky's office. We never told, but at one point we were discovered looking at the magazines and that was the end of the Helpers Club.

## 23 The Register

There were not many warm rooms at Linden Hall. It was an old school that was dark in both color and design. As a ninth-grade freshman, I shared a room with two other girls. Our rooms were meant for study and dressing. These rooms were especially stark in color and décor. It was, of course, Amish country and I assume the design was influenced by the locals. We were not allowed to talk to the locals when we met them on the street, which amplified the coldness I experienced in the rooms of their fashioning. Maybe there was a bit of passive aggression on the part of the school's leadership here: *If the Linden Hall girls were too good to talk to us, we will make their lives, inside those walls, less than inviting.*

We slept in dormitories. Our privacy was protected by the walls of our individual alcoves. Everything about this new home was chilling. And, as winter approached and my body was shrinking, I felt an even greater need to seek out warmth. Outside of my room was a floor grid through which heat rose in strong waves. Everyone referred to it as the "*register*." It was my favorite place in the building. It was the only place that I felt warm and cared for. Until I was called away to do school things, I stood fixed, over my register. And, it became known, by students and housemothers, as "*Dicki's register*."

The thinner I got, the more I found that students, especially older students, would congregate around me and my register. For the first time, I was the youngest, and becoming, the smallest. Upon my register, I stood, receiving my nurturance from the heat below me and the attention around me. It was my throne, and I was the princess that I always wanted to be, the one who was cared for. This was different from the princess of my mother's home, the princess who was a *Queen in the making,* anointed with all household and caregiving tasks fit for the Queen. I was Cinderella when at home. Here I was someone new. I was creating her. She would be adored and cared for. Everyone seemed concerned for my well-being. They wanted me to eat. I wanted to stay small so I could continue to have their attention.

I think that the heat from the register moving up and through me provided a warmth like food does when you eat. I felt full after a register fix. The fullness I felt eating a big meal made me feel weighed down. The register's heat made me feel light and almost euphoric. I could stay there all day, basking in this light. It was much better than a fast quick meal whose duration I would never choose to extend.

## 24 The First Princess Room

We moved to the big house on the big road between East Hampton and Amagansett. I was in second grade and Mom was pregnant with Randy. He was born a few months after we moved in. Now there were six of us children. The tiny house on the tiny street had been home to us for three and a half years. During that time our family grew to include three more children and two dogs. Mamie, our black lab must have missed that place. She was better at letting everyone know what mattered to her than were we. Every day she would leave the new house on the big road and every night Daddy Tom would drive over there and pick her up. She would be sitting on the lawn waiting to go inside. I thought it was sad that we didn't really say goodbye to our tiny house. We arrived at the new big house on the big road, and everything was set up clean and new with no reminders of what we had left behind. A fresh paint job and new furniture can hide all the secrets.

The new house was the place where my Princess apprenticeship began. I was in training to take on the role of Princess Perfect. I was the chosen child to carry Mom's legacy. I did not know what that meant yet, only that I was the only child to have her own room. It was perfectly set up when I arrived. A double bed with a canopy and lace took up a good part of space. A matched set of dressers, one tall and one wide with an attached mirror were there as well. Two bedside tables flanked the bed. I remember wondering why I had all that furniture, and my siblings did not. It seemed that my room was the show place. A token. All effort put into making it look just right. The proper room for the chosen princess. I was alone in that room on that first day. I was alone in that room for most days. When I opened my new closet, I found a brand-new navy-blue sailor dress. I wondered where my old clothes were. I missed them. This was my dress for going to second grade. That I looked the part seemed important.[8] I was not sure what the part was, but it was a part that I thought was necessary to take on. Mom reminded me that I should tell people, if they asked, that my last name was *Strong*. She did not want people to know that she had been married twice, so I could not tell my true last name which was *Johnson*. The lie did not make sense because I know that my name was *Johnson* in school. I think about why mom was embarrassed to admit she had been married twice. Somehow it must have tainted her image, or the one she wanted to have people see. And I must have been part of that image. What others saw, or what she wanted them to see, was different from the people we were at home. I don't remember every having her ask what I thought or wanted. Actually, I don't remember conversations with anyone at home. I only see rooms and the objects in those rooms. Maybe I developed relationships with things and with animals, both of which Mom seemed to value more than the children. From my room with its perfect arrangement and my closet with the one dress, I hear the others running around wildly. Unspoken was the rule that I alone, could not run around wildly. For the time being, I knew how to behave. I don't remember being told what that entailed, but in elementary school I was good because I wanted Mom to be proud of me. I think that was it. Something else about my room: It had two doors. It was a square room that was positioned between two perpendicular hallways. Later on, the wildness from which my room had been insulated, consumed it like flames. My brothers and sisters and all the dogs used it as a breezeway for their free form antics. In my absence, there was no need for sanction. Whatever image I and my room were to uphold had been forsaken, and no one was willing to take over that part. Only I had been groomed to carry it. The princess room, with no princess in it, became a highway for a lot of fast-moving children.

## 25 Individual Photos

There were not many photographs of us as children. Cameras were not everyday props as there were no handheld phones in the 1960's. The pictures from my childhood, the pictures of me with my siblings were the staged Christmas pictures that mom arranged to have taken. For a while they were taken in Pennsylvania by her parents' photographer. That meant we were packed up in the station wagon and driven the long six-hour haul through the mountains for that one captured image that somehow connected her with her parents. I'm sure there were local photographers that could have come to our own house and taken our photograph. Later on, by the time Randy (number six) was born, the Christmas picture was staged in our own living room. By that time her parents were gone. There was no longer a need for my mom to impress them. Mom was the youngest of ten children most of whom were much older than she. She grew up with a brother who was close in age to her. I have a photo of her with that brother Philip taken by the famed photographer Bachrach in Pennsylvania. That must have been their Christmas picture. I assume that, as mom seemed compelled to have her children's annual image captured by that same photographer, or at least the same studio.

Other than that, there were no pictures of us that I can remember. Just as there were no conversations between two of us. I don't remember discussing anything with my siblings or with my mother. A photo taken of one of us solo would have been a conversation between the person with the camera and her subject. It seems that the value of those group shots was not in the conversation, in the process of engaging. Rather the end product, a statement of proof. What was it that my mother needed to prove? And to whom?? I think it was to her father. She spoke of him with admiration. Of her mother she said little. I do remember her saying that she remembered her only as old and sedentary. Her father was active and photos from her childhood, the few, were with him. She may have been competing with her mom to outdo the number of offspring she had produced. Mom almost made it. She did have ten pregnancies although only seven children survived.

We were not taught to have individual relationships with her or with each other. She could not teach us what she had not known herself. It was not that they were denied to us; it was just not part of our daily diet.

I looked for pictures of myself as a child. I first remember thinking about the lack of them when I was ten or eleven. It was stunning to me to see a photo of myself, of me alone on the beach in Eagles Mere, where we spent half of every childhood summer with my father and my half siblings. There, on Daddy's Pennsylvania office desk, was a picture of me, all alone me. He had taken the

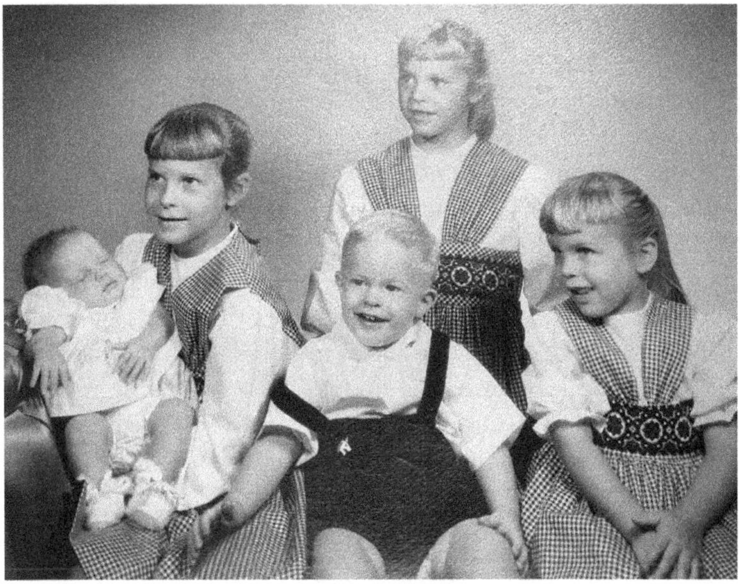

FIGURE 13 Christmas with five children, 1959

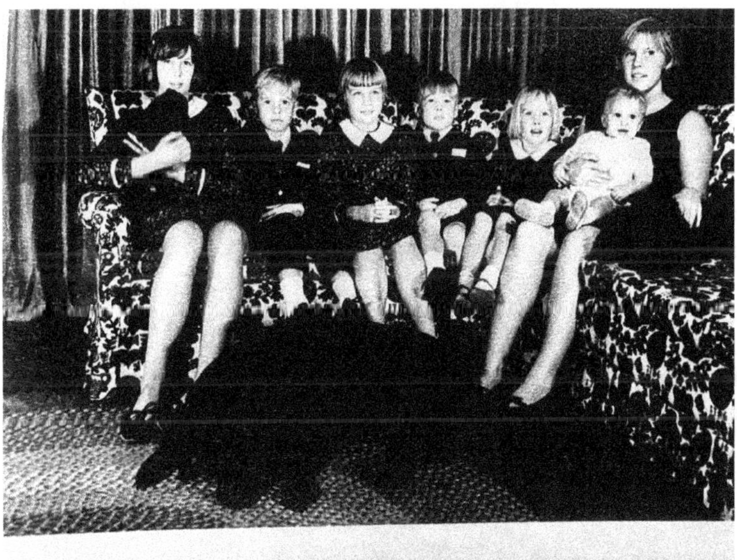

FIGURE 14 Christmas with seven children, 1965

time to have a conversation with me, the conversation needed between two people to produce the photographic image. I was stunned as it made evident to me the lack of such pictures of me, or of any of mom's children in her home.

## 26 The Baby Carriage

My fifth birthday was a milestone for me. My favorite gift was a half-slip which housed within the periphery of its baseline circle, an inflatable tube. It was made so that one could inflate the circle to create a slip with a wide bottom, a hoop skirt. When you blew up the bottom it looked like the skirt that Cinderella wore when she went to the prince's party. When I put it on, I felt grownup: "I can't believe that I made it this far. I am five years old." This is what I remember about my fifth year.

It is small wonder that I felt so grownup at five. I was the eldest of all my siblings, so was, as you know, expected to do a fair amount of caretaking. Perception is all relative: at the top of the chronological pyramid, compared to my baby brothers and sisters, I did seem to be mature. There is a photograph of me pushing my brother Randy in his baby carriage on Newtown Lane in East Hampton. That was a distance, at least a mile, from our house. I was put

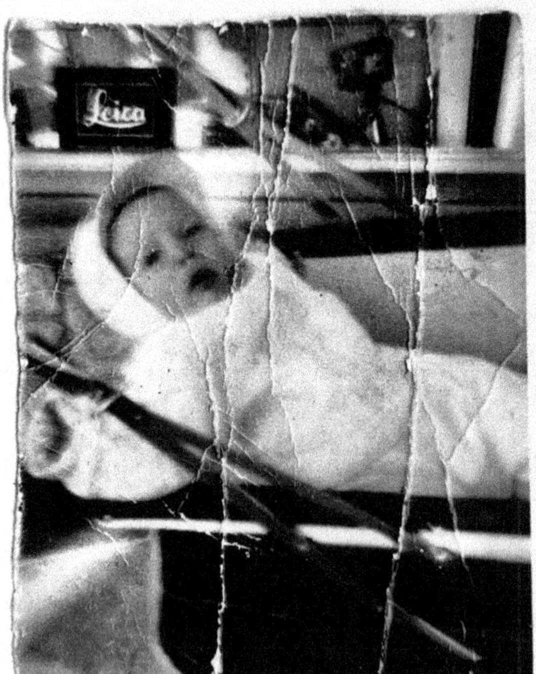


FIGURE 15 Baby Randy by Starlight Camera, 1960

in the position of being responsible for a baby, at seven years of age. I took the picture. It was the only picture there was of Randy as a baby.

Photos became a form of talking to each other. The photographs that my siblings and I took of each other showed everyday life, not posed and fancy-dressed Christmas card pictures.

A bit more about the camera. It was a Brownie Starlight. I bought it with my babysitting money that I had saved from my babysitting gig with Andrew Reed. Andrew's father was a Manhattan artist who had moved his family away from the city into the country. East Hampton was friendly back then, and stores were owned by locals. This was before all the big names moved in and took away all the local stores. This was before it became a place for Ralph Lauren, Tiffany's and all those other New York City stores. This was before it became known as *The Hamptons*. So, Paul Reed bought a little store which became Reed's Photography. I am not sure whether I came to know the family through the shop or after I began babysitting. I think my mom told him that I would be a good babysitter for his son. As she had already consigned me to that role with my sibs, it made sense that she might offer me up. Andrew was four years old, and I was nine years old. It may seem odd for a girl to be babysitting a kid that was just five years younger than her. But when it was happening, it seemed normal. I had heard, a few years later, that in parts of Africa where many adults had died of AIDS, the oldest kids had to take charge of all the younger ones. The average age of these head of household was nine years. So, who was I to see myself as having to do too much, when all I had to do was care for one child? And, as a benefit, I bought my Brownie Starlight, took photos of my siblings, sometimes one at a time, and was given a discount to process the film by Mr. Reed.

When I was twelve, I had not yet gone through puberty. My physical body was still childlike. It housed an emotional body that had taken on many adult responsibilities. I was standing in the dressing room preparing for my ballet class. Looking in the mirror, I noticed that one of my hips appeared to be higher than the other and the shoulder on the opposite side of my body seemed lifted out of balance with the other. I would adjust them both manually into proper placement with their other side. Later I read that scoliosis develops in girls when there is an imbalance between the development of their physical and their emotional bodies. The disharmony between the two produces a curvature in the spine. I always thought it was normal to have to make this manual adjustment and found out later, through x-rays, that I had a significant scoliosis. X-Rays were photographs that told the truth. You can't pose with fancy clothes or fake smiles for an x-ray. The truth was that my body was showing on the outside what was happening inside to my heart and my mind.

## 27 Grooming

There are more photographs in our home of Mom than of us children. Except for the annual posed Christmas picture, there is little that freezes those moments of kids actually playing together. Did we play together? I think that the image of *posing* holds significance. As appearances seemed to be highly valued, photographs depicted that which was of most esteemed. Mom's photos were of her as either an equestrian or a debutante. She is holding a trophy, standing beside her horse, or leaping over a wall in a competition. These images remind her of and convey to us, her status as elite, as a winner. She was groomed to be one of the chosen. Here in our home away from her origins, maybe debutantes and equestrians are of little consequence.

I do know that the social hierarchy in horse cultures places riding "English" at the top and riding "Western" at the bottom. In Pennsylvania, and especially at Linden Hall (where she was equestrian royalty[9] having competed in and mastered the art of dressage), only English saddles were acceptable. However, here in East Hampton the locals had a riding club, The Trailblazers, which mom joined. Saddles were all western there. Clearly a step down. Maybe that is why all the posed pictures of mom present her as the royal that she was.

Our backyard became the horse pasture when we acquired our two quarter horses. These are smaller than the thoroughbreds that mom grew up with but horses that were sturdy and most able to accommodate the western saddles. "Parley" was mom's horse. He had been abused by a former owner and it was only mom whom he would let get near to or ride him. "Bright Eyes" was the kids' and Daddy's horse. We took turns riding her.

When I was in seventh grade a handsome young man, a high school teacher moved into town. I am not sure how Mom came to know him, but I do remember that he became a member of the Trailblazer's Club. There may have been rides in the woods that he shared with Mom. What I do know is that, at some point, I was sharing rides with him in the woods. He was able to handle "Parley." He may have been the only other human, bedsides Mom that could do so. Maybe Mom groomed him to assume that position. Maybe she was grooming me to assume some position that I did not understand at the time. On our rides in the woods there came a time when the handsome teacher would stop and lean over to kiss me. On the lips. I did not think at the time that that was a bad thing. He did tell me that it should be our secret. Later that year he confided in me that he had met a woman and was going to marry her. He also confided that when they got older, he would leave her and come for me. When I was old enough.

Looking back now I wonder if this was still another attempt to have me assume my mom's crown. Had she, in. fact, been involved romantically with

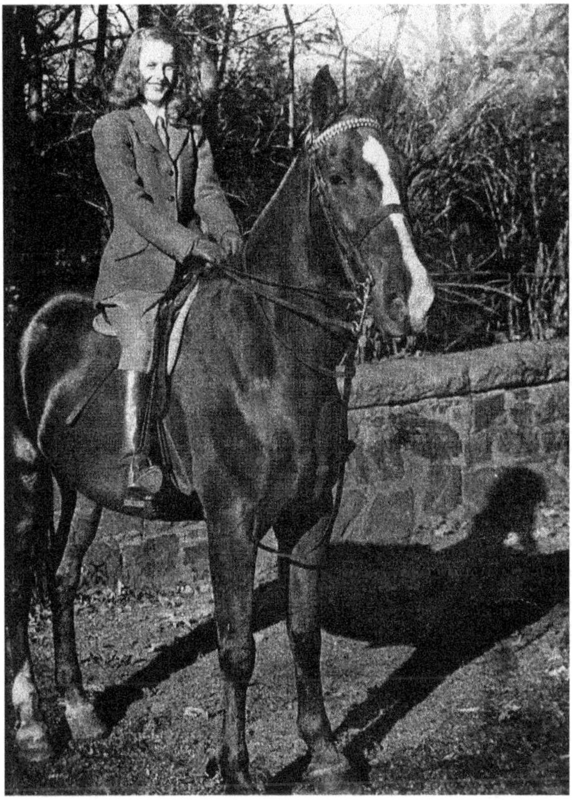

FIGURE 16 Mom on horseback, 1947

this young teacher? Was she positioning me to assume a role that she could not? Did she know that he was kissing me in the woods and, if so, did she experience some vicarious benefit? When I stopped eating at Linden Hall and needed to come home, Mom had this young teacher, who also was a pilot, and has a small two-seater plane, pick me up and fly me home. He did not try to kiss me on that return journey.

## 28 Fruitwood Table

Celebrating birthdays was something that all kids got to do. Even if you were Presbyterian, you had a special day that was all yours, every year. Most special celebrations, I have thought, were created for Catholic or Jewish kids. So, as a boring Presbyterian, I was happy that birthdays were for us too.

My twelfth birthday was on a Friday night and all my best friends came over to have dinner and cake. Mom made her special German Chocolate cake for me, and Daddy Tom made us spaghetti and meatballs. Barb, Chelle, Shelley, Toni, Donna, and Sally Story were my best friends then, so they were all there. Because it was my birthday, we got to sit in the dining room around Mom's special fruitwood table. It was special because it was one of the objects that she inherited from her parents or from her grandparents. She always talked about the special things that came from her family and would be passed down to us when she died.

There was one problem. Sally Story was Catholic and Catholics had a special Catholic practice for Fridays. On Friday they were not allowed to eat meat. Not eating meat made them feel purer and more religious. This practice, that was for Catholics only, made them seem even more special to me than they already were in my eyes. Everything about their religion seemed magical to me. They had all kinds of rituals. Some seemed majestic and others seemed difficult. I liked the idea of saying "No" to food that you really like. I was so impressed that Sally watched us all eat our meatballs, and just smiled. She seemed really strong but also really devout. I heard that word even in my Presbyterian church.

I decided that I would secretly follow the Catholic rule of not eating meat on Fridays. I also decided that I wanted to wear a yarmulke like the Jewish men wear in their temple (that is the Jewish church) and only open one present a day over Christmas rather than all at once on one day. I wanted to belong to

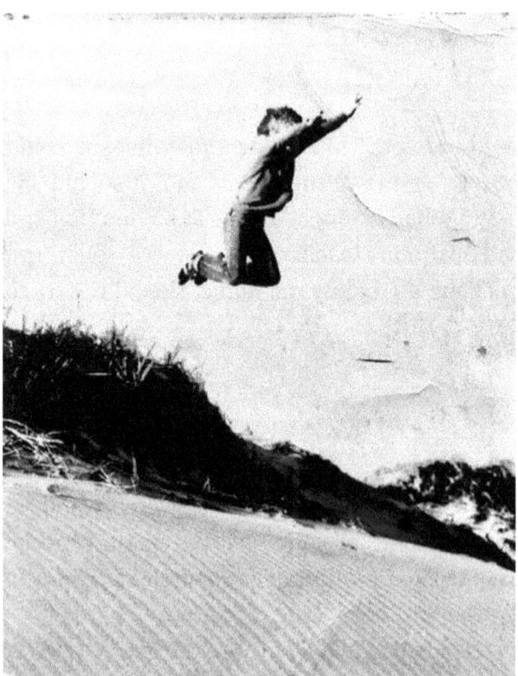

FIGURE 17 Billy leaping on Main Beach, 1969

a religion that had special rituals. If I could not be Catholic or Jewish, I would borrow some of their special practices and make them my own. No more eating meat on Fridays. I wondered if there was other food that I might stop eating to feel purer and more special. I would think about that later.

The Main Beach in East Hampton is where we spent most of our summers. It was the place where the local community gathered. It was our outdoor together place; The church was our inside place. Most of my community memories were set in one of the two arenas. A boardwalk connected the pavilion, where all was dry, with the beach, almost to the high tide mark of the ocean. Jumping from the base of the boardwalk to the sand, one entered what I experienced as *Center Stage*. When we first moved to this town, I see me jumping with my sister into it. I was two and a half and my sister was a year younger. We were toddlers dressed in matching dresses. In the beginning our costumes were perfect. We were the new family with the presence of aristocracy. Center Stage, Main Beach is where all opening acts were presented. After we had been in town for a while, and after mom had remarried and had a few more children, there was no need for opening night costumes.

To the right of Center Stage was the area where all the mothers collected. With their beach chairs, straw flower sun hats, white noses, movie magazines and coolers with food for their children, they set up camp for the day. Mostly the children were elsewhere, either center or to the left of it. We would move up and down the boardwalk, finding treasures in the food court or in someone's changing locker. It seemed to me that we were always moving up and down and finally, when it was too hot, into the ocean we dove. In the water we were at home. Her sea womb was familiar, reminiscent. To the left, I feel threat, the unfamiliar. It was like the feeling of being out in the sunshine of day and when looking left, feeling the draw of the dark forest. Moving in that direction always meant taking a risk. With that risk we might find something never before seen or experienced. Not many people hung out on that side. It was a journey place. It was the direction of west toward rocky jetties. I once ventured that way and found hidden caves in the jetties. The parents always warned us to not go there. As children this warning was also an enticement.

When I was a teenager, or maybe a preteen, most of my beach time was spent walking west, away from the sun. I was not much of a beach sitter, or a tanning type of girl. Later, in high school we would hang out at night on the beach, with a center stage bonfire. I found out one Monday, during school, that my boyfriend was drawn left, away from the bonfire, by another girl. This was my first heartbreak. My boyfriend wrote me a confessional note begging my forgiveness. Of course, he blamed the girl for his betrayal. I still have that note, from 1968, in my Revised Standard Version of my New Testament bible.

Something else that is important about the beach and going left is this: A memory. I am running down the boardwalk, and just as I am about to leap off, I veer left. The wind catches me and I am lifted from vertical to horizontal. Arms out-stretched, I feel myself flying. I shift my body and can control my direction. The memory is so precise, I can feel the flight in my body as I envision it. I have asked my childhood friends and my siblings if they remember doing the same. No one yet has shared this jump into flight that is so vivid for me. I am not sure what it means. It could be a dream, but one so real that I am determined that it happened. I think about going back there and trying it now, just to see. I am not writing about dreams. That will be another chapter. I am convinced that the experience was real. Now, there are so many people inhabiting my childhood beach. The city people have changed the town and the beach with their money. They have no use for the community, for the distinction between center, right and left. There is no longer any place to jump, fly, or land. The mysterious pathway left is now a clutter of very expensive beach cabanas. What were once undulating dunes with blades of long beach grass, now hold secure, "private, no trespassing" signs. When we were young, we flew from those dunes and rode our horses through them without restriction or saddle.

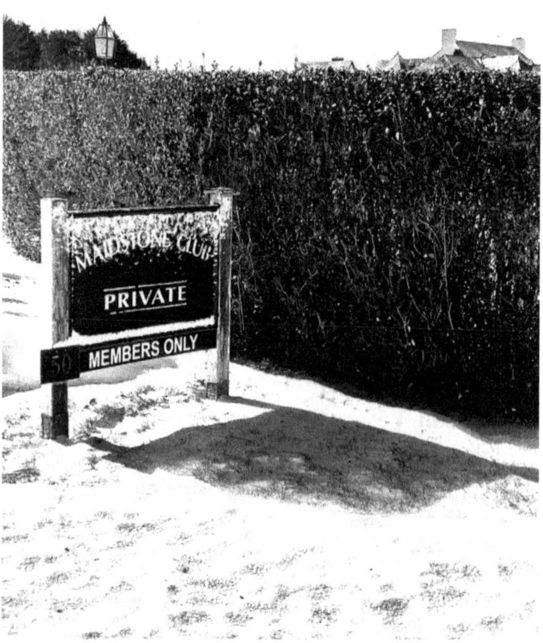


FIGURE 18 Maidstone club is private

## 29 Townie or Country Club Set

Really, I did not belong in either group. Although we lived in the town as locals, we were nouveau locals having no heritage there. We never quite qualified for the country club set. Mom worked at obtaining entre into the club set, flashing her debutante and dressage credentials. Her presentation was not quite enough. For one thing, she had too many children. Families with more than six children were seen as either Catholic, out of control, or lower class of some variety.

Back in Pennsylvania, she was an aristocrat, but I think the rules of engagement were different here in New York. And then she married a local, which in caste and class system measurements, placed her in the lower rung.

When her parents died and left her a substantial inheritance, she went mansion house hunting. There were six children at that point, and she was looking for something amazing that was close to the ocean. A private association area fit the bill; the house was perfect and within walking distance to the beach. But our family was not perfect. The association did not allow Jewish, Latin, or Black families or those with more than five children. I think this was the first time I really experienced being seen as marginalized. Racism and classism were surely intact there, but we had never been specifically called out or placed directly below the dominant select group. I think Mom tried even harder the to prove she was groomed with "proper breeding." She instilled in us the necessity to always look and act the part.[10] We did finally find a great house. Next door the Brady's lived. They were Catholic and had twelve children.

The house was on the right side of town. Poor white or all Black families lived "under the bridge." I don't remember being told of that division but somehow it was communicated. A few of my friends live "under the bridge." Now that I think of it, they were not WASPS but rather Italian or Jewish. Both friends had parents that had their own businesses, one a clothing store, the other an electronics repair shop. The families lived above their downstairs businesses. And we lived on the other side of the bridge but were not eligible to join the clubs open to the elite. I think it was more than the number of children that kept us out. Maybe it was because my stepfather was a local, a townie. But because Mom was not, we were often excluded from townie activities. As a child, in kindergarten and elementary school, I did not feel excluded. I went to public school and was surrounded by cousins and other locals. As kids we had not yet learned about classism or segregation. We all played with each other. It was what I observed in my mother's behaviors that set the stage for understanding exclusion and the need for putting on airs. Over time all that subliminal suggestion caught up with me. There was no real place that I belonged, no group that I was truly a part of. We were immigrants is a town that had only two castes: Townie or Country Club Set. Everyone else aspired to be one or the other.

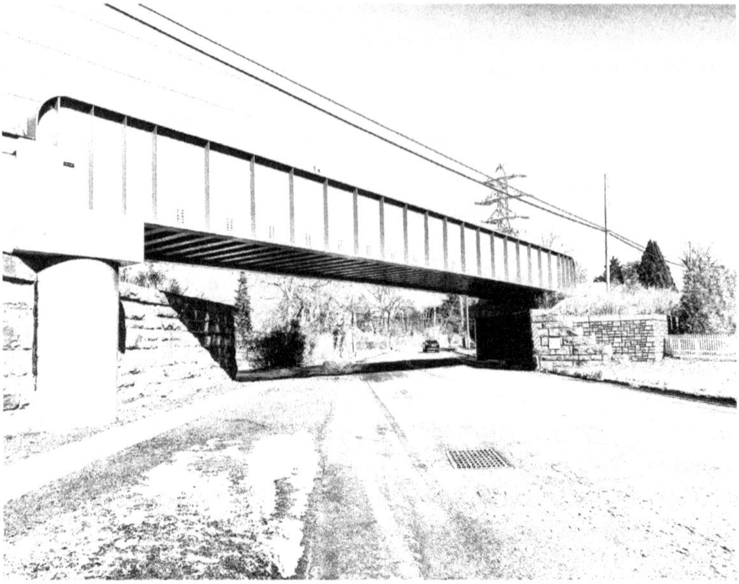

FIGURE 19 Under the bridge

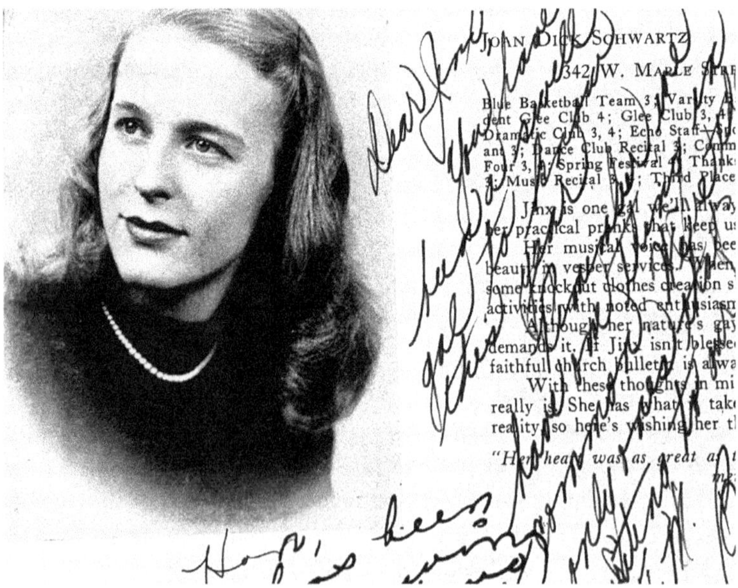


FIGURE 20 Jinx: Linden Hall yearbook

When Mom was in high school and College, so her story goes, she was given the nickname "Jinx." As she tells it, she had so many boyfriends that she was said to Jinx them. I think that meant that she put a spell on each of them. She made each believe that she was true to only him. In other words, she was living a lie. In her telling of this story to us, she spoke with pride rather than shame. In her story, Jinx was going steady with five boys at the same time. Because both her high school and college were private girls' schools, she could get away with pulling the wool over multiple boys' eyes simultaneously: She just had to remember to wear the correct going steady ring when visiting the respective boy at his school.

This story was important because it represented to me what she valued. I wonder if she rebelled against the script handed to her as a woman. I wonder if this rebellion was against patriarchal values and against men in general. She seemed to be telling us that if you are pretty enough and smart enough, you can outsmart men at their own game. This was a confusing story to me as a little girl. Mom was so blond and pretty and I know that I wanted to be like her.

Maybe playing all that Bacharach music whose lyrics subliminally enforced the loyal wife script was a defense mechanism. Maybe it helped to keep the rebel that she truly was in check.[11] I think of that music often as it also shaped my thinking about what was in store for me when I moved into the realm of womanhood. Mostly my coming of age was being shaped by the conflicts between truths and lies. I wanted to be like Mom, but I was not sure which part of her presentation I wanted to mimic.[12] She was beautiful, athletic, and musical. However, as I grew into consciousness (this did not happen until I was living away from home), I was able to stand back and see that the world she wanted everyone to see her in was mostly make believe. It became harder and harder to know what was true and what she had made up. She had attempted to jinx us all, even her children.

## 30 Clean Plate Club

I should mention, or put into historical perspective, my launching. My parents lived through WWII. Daddy was in the Navy, an officer, and could have been a career – officer but opted to step down so he could be home with his anticipated family. He was born in 1919 and came home from the war and married young Mom, who was ten years his junior. As her story goes, her true love Mac, died in the war and Daddy was a golf buddy of her favorite brother-in-law. The family thought him to be a perfect partner and guardian to the young Jinx. Theirs was a magnificent story book wedding. I was born in 1952, and my sister in 1953. My parents divorced in 1954, or at least my mother left at that point. She moved to East Hampton, a summer resort where her parents had summered. I think they set her up with a house and car there. My half sibs were born in 1956, 1958, 1959, 1960 and 1965. That will place us all in time.

I think that there must have been restriction on food allowances or access during the war because, all children of the 50's that I have known, were members of the "clean plate club." That is what having to eat everything presented on our plates was called in our house. We were not allowed to leave the table, at my mother or my father's homes, until every morsel was consumed. I do remember hearing reminders at the table that there were "starving children somewhere in the world" and this was reasoned to be the explanation for why we must eat all of our food. I never understood how stuffing my own body would in any way help starving children in other countries.

There were two times that stand out for me as times I was forced to stay at the table until I had eaten everything. Both times I was determined not to eat those foods left and undesirable. This might have been the beginning of my relationship with food and exerting my own control over what I put into my body. It reminds me of having some choice in what one might plant in the earth. The first experience was in Mom's home. I was left at the table staring at a plate of bay scallops. The smell was enough to make me gag. I knew that I could not eat them. When my parents left the room (I think I might have been left there for hours), I stuffed them into my pants pocket. I was released from my stronghold when my parents returned to find my plate empty. I think I was five years old and didn't have much foresight. My pants went through the washer releasing the ocean of scallops into the basin. When my mom discovered the mess, of course, I was punished.

The second time was at my father's house and was not dissimilar. This time it was a disgusting plate of stewed tomatoes. They were slimy and the smell made me almost throw up. I do remember sitting at the table alone for what seemed like the whole night. No one came to release me, and I do not remember ever eating them. There was no way to hide stewed tomatoes like I did with the scallops. What I do remember is my daddy being angry and then leaving me alone. Neither of us wanted to give in, but parents always win, and kids are forced to eat things that make them feel sick.[13]

## 31 Kotex 1945

The time to learn about becoming a woman, at least the physical woman, was sixth grade. In our classroom the girls were taken to the music room and shown a film about getting your period. It was sponsored by Kotex, the popular sanitary pad company at that time. It was very matter of fact, with not any mention of the emotional transition we as little girls might experience.[14] I thought that maybe Mom would be able to share some insight that might help me understand what this *period* was all about.

She did not have much to say. For someone who talked so much about her unique experiences as a beautiful teenager, her sharing of experiences that might bond us rather than separate us was minimal. I guess she talked about what was important to her. I think her mother didn't talk to her about becoming a woman so maybe she didn't know how to tell me. Identity was created by what she observed, not by what she was gifted. At any rate, I remember that Mom's response to my questions about getting my period was to give me a booklet, also published by Kotex. It was probably one she had been given as a teenager as the girls in the booklet were wearing clothes from the 40's and were engaged in activities that didn't seem modern. My guess was that this was the booklet she had been given to explain menstruation. It was probably easier for her to let the book tell me what I needed to know than it was for her to engage in conversation about the life change and how that might impact my identity. I didn't think much about it at the time, other than to think the clothes and the hairdos of the models were definitely from another time. The fact that she had saved her period book and gave it to me, made me feel close to her in a way. At least that was something we shared. I guess that most of what she told us about her own growing up was dramatized. She worshipped her father and when we asked her about her mother, she said that "she was always old." I think she was raised by maids and didn't feel too much love from her mother. Mom did not know how to be a mother. She did know how to be pretty and get attention for that. She shared with me what it meant to become a woman as it was shared with her. I can only imagine because her parents and all her siblings are all gone and can't tell me anything about their childhoods. Mom is also gone. My knowledge of that time comes from my memory of it and what of that memory stood out as unique moments and images. I remember the Kotex book and how I hoped to get my period so that I could belong to the community of women. Most of my friends did, in fact, get theirs soon after the movie. It took me several more years to belong. And when it finally came, I felt confused. I had thought I would feel really great. Rather, I was not sure to which group I wanted to belong. I never did seem to be truly part of any group, having been forced to pretend from an early age. I think the period brought with it a desire to return to the children's group, to belong with my younger siblings. Mom had not made it clear what becoming a woman would involve. All that I understood at that time was what she showed by her actions. I was learning that being a woman meant telling a lot of lies and acting in a way that would make me acceptable. My period revealed to me a distinction between truth and pretense. How you look is not always how you feel.

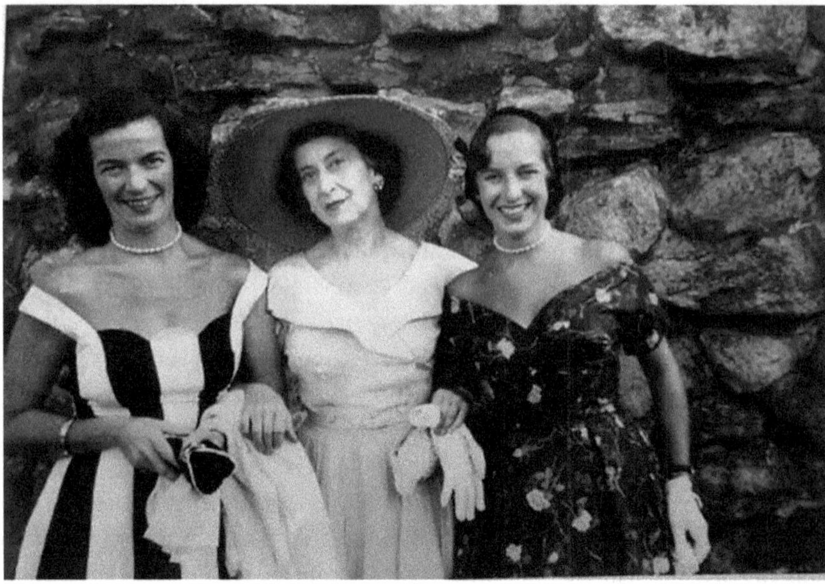

FIGURE 21 Marmie and her daughters, 1945

## 32 Barbizon Hotel

Two of Mom's books fascinated me. She had studied to be both a debutante and a medical assistant of some kind. There was a medical book that displayed real photographs of all sorts of deformities and skin conditions. I remember sneaking the book out of her drawer and hiding in a closet to look at the pictures. They were horrific. I could not, for some reason, get enough. Children were not supposed to be exposed to those things hidden. I was never quite sure what was to be hidden from kids and what, exactly, all those things hidden from us had in common. I did know that we were not supposed to look at that medical book. I think that what adults chose for us to see had to be pretty, which made it acceptable. At any rate, at eight, I was captivated by this book that showed me that not everything was as it appeared. My sisters were also interested in this book. We were determined to learn about all those things that our parents would not tell us about.

Later, another hidden book was a Victorian novel by "Anonymous." This was not one of Mom's books. One of us found it while babysitting somewhere. I don't think it was me rather one of my friends found it and passed it around to all of us eighth grade girls. It described in detail, every possible sex act with every kind of living creature. It was a 600-page book. I remember going up to the attic, another hiding place, to read it. About halfway through, I decided that I should not read anymore because, as a virgin, I had no experience with sex. I was amazed that I had such a sense of self-control and a sense of how stories, pictures, music, and films, might influence me badly. I thought that reading the book would jade me in a way that I would come to consider the acts described to be normal.

The other of Mom's books that I loved leafing through was one that she allowed us to indulge in. However, it was delicate, so we were only able to physically hold it in her presence. It was her scrap book from her high school and college years. There were flattened corsages, western union telegrams, coasters from Manhattan restaurants, train schedules, Barbizon hotel bills, and match covers. We were told about her adventures while she was at Briarcliff Manor, a college about one hour north of Manhattan. She and her girlfriends would take the train into the city to meet their respective boyfriends who were cadets at West Point Academy, which was also close to the city. Her boyfriend was Mac. He later died in the war.

The girls, as we understood it, had to stay at the Barbizon on an all-girls floor. That was the respectable way to be in those days. Her adventures sounded so exciting. I imagined her dressing in beautiful clothes; there were pictures of her in those outfits. She seemed to live such a glamorous life. Remember, she told us that she was "going steady" with five boys at the same time, at one point. I think this was not that time, as Mac seemed to be the only one whose telegrams and dating relics were in her scrap book. I thought that I would never become a girl who had enough adventures to fill a scrapbook with its details. I was in middle school at this point, and not very glamourous. Later I wondered why, in her life as a wife and mother, she never left her home on Long Island. Manhattan was 100 miles away and she never went there. Also, she never had a passport and only went away, to Florida, on her honeymoon. I wondered why she became so isolated and chose not to explore and venture away as she had before she was married. It reminded me of what I imagined the Burt Bacharach music did for her. It helped to keep her restricted. It reminded her of what she must appear to be. I know that how she presented herself to the social community was not her whole story. The hidden was like the medical book. Truths not acceptable needed to be kept quiet.

## 33 Cinnamon

Cinnamon was meant for oatmeal, and, at Marmie's house, there was always oatmeal. Daddy Bill (this is what we called my father) sat with us for breakfast. The bowls were placed on the table with spoons and napkins. The oatmeal

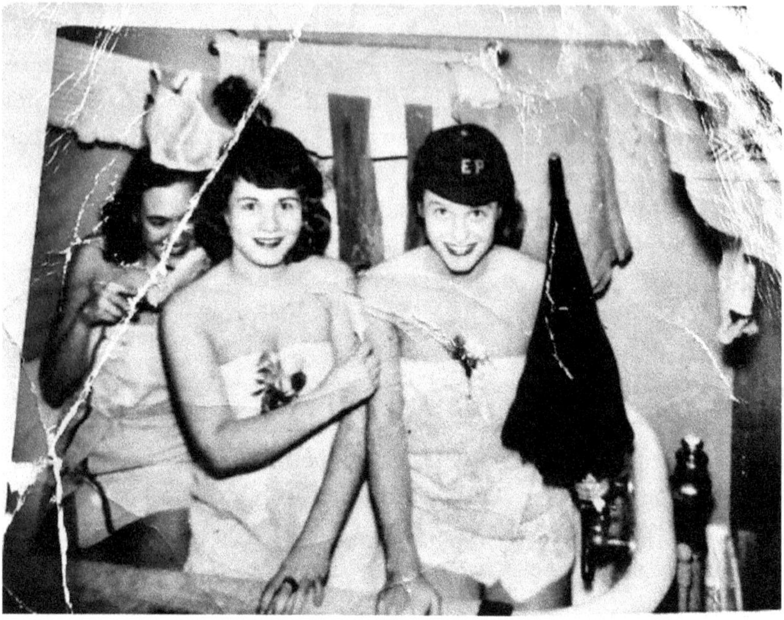

FIGURE 22 Preparing for her date, 1948

must have been prepared before we woke. Marmie had lots of chores for us to do before we could go to the lake, so the oatmeal had to be ready to send us off. This strange damp house nurtured us all. *All* are the many cousins, moms, and aunts, by day, uncles and dads by night. Dads go off to work while the moms and kids do "Marmie" work and go to the lake. Marmie believed that it was important to raise us with a sense of ethical service; I think that might be the term. She came up with the strangest of jobs for us cousins: painting her back porch step (we ran out of one-color paint, and she gave us a completely different color to paint the last few risers). Pulling out all the ferns that laced the foundation of her large Queen Ann style home was a favorite Marmie chore. Another time she gave us a plastic pool that she wanted to make into a fishpond. The site for the proposed pool was a rock formation. I think we were on that job for many days as we could not dig through rock.

Daddy Bill had to go to work which was about an hour from Marmie's summer house. I was always so happy that he sat with us, that he gave us his time while we ate our oatmeal. Mom, back home, did not sit with us while we ate breakfast. In fact, I don't remember breakfast at her home. Let me clarify who the moms are: my biological father and Mom divorced when I was two, so my sister and I would spend half the summer with my father and my stepmom at Marmie's. Marmie is my father's mom.

Back to the cinnamon. Mom only cooked holiday meals and had a few specialties: German Chocolate cake, German stuffing, German Potato salad, and corn pudding. She was big on German everything. I think this was because her family passed down certain recipes but did not actually pass down the experience of being together and preparing them. All was remembered as a written recipe. Her own mom was very old and probably did not cook with or for her. In her parents' home there were people hired to cook and attend to her. I don't think that she had oatmeal as a child because she only gave us, her children, Coco Krispies and Capt'n Crunch. Those breakfasts we could serve to ourselves.

Even though we had strange chores at Marmie's, we also had oatmeal that someone took the time to prepare for us.

## 34 Knitting

Mom was a fabulous knitter. I am not sure who taught her to knit because her mother was really old when Mom was growing up. Maybe her housekeeper taught her. Mom was not one of those moms that baked cookies and hung out with her kids. Her stories were not about growing up with her own sisters and brothers but about all her boyfriends. In fact, she never talked about her childhood except to tell us how wonderful and handsome her father was. I know that someone baked cookies when she was a girl because, when her parents died, she inherited their cookie jar, which was a ceramic pig. I think her housekeeper, whom she did mention a bit, must have baked cookies. Back to the knitting.

Mom did not teach us to knit or to do much of anything like that. I learned to sew and to cook from recipes in 7th grade home economics class. All the girls in middle school were required to take home ec. I was glad to have someone to teach me because later, I made my own clothes after mom lost interest in dressing me up. When I was visiting my father's house in Pennsylvania, my step grandmother, Grandma Koogle taught me to crochet. After that I made a lot of crocheted things, mostly hats and scarves for presents. It was nice to have this skill. It was also nice to have a grandmother to teach me things. Mom's parents died when I was in elementary school, so I did not have much time with them. All I remember of them was their house which was across the street from a cemetery and had an elevator in it. Daddy Bill's mom, Marmie, was an actress who married my grandfather, who was older and a Federal Supreme Court judge and was fired for taking bribes. There are several buildings at Bucknell that are named for him. Mom told us that he died of "chronic meanness."

Here is what Mom was proud of: (1) her many boyfriends, (2) her beautiful singing voice, (3) her thick blond hair, (4) her thin figure, and (5) having so many babies that she almost outdid her mother. My grandmother had ten children; Mom had seven but insisted that she had ten pregnancies and lost a few babies through miscarriages. Knitting was maybe the only domestic skill that she shared with us. The sharing was an exhibition of her skill rather than a teaching and passing on of the skill. I learned how to knit in high school but don't know who taught me. Years later I watched a local homeless woman knit a sweater around her body thorough out the fall. It kept her warm in the winter. In the spring she unraveled it.

## 35 Cinderella

Cinderella was my favorite Disney princess. I think she was my favorite because no one knew she was a princess. She was a princess in hiding. She was the princess that I wanted to be. It was all pretty confusing, this princess thing. Mom was gorgeous and had never been a princess in hiding. She was always standing on the front line, fully adorned with perfectly matching blond clothes and jewelry. Sometimes she was even asked to model for the local clothing boutiques. In East Hampton this was a big deal because it was a tourist town and lots of people from the city came to the fashion shows. One time I was even in a fashion show with her, modeling kids' clothes for Abercrombie and Fitch. I was pretty by my association with her. The runway was never my comfort zone. I was never blond, and blond was the way to be back then.

Cinderella did not speak much but knew how to sew and do alone things. She needed no adornment or fancy clothes to be a princess in hiding. I was not flashy either. I see myself as like Cinderella because I withdrew from the mainstream and chose not to compete with the really pretty girls. Mom wanted me to be one of those pretty girls who was always front and center and that is why, for a while, she dressed me up to look like them. I know that I wanted to please her and sometimes, even to look like her. One year, when I was about eight years old, I started setting my hair in curlers and had little flippy waves above my eyebrows. I fixed my hair to look just like mom's 60s do. I was trying hard to be like her, but I looked like a baby dressing up in mommy clothes. I was confused, I think, over which princess I should be. I wanted to be the princess in hiding, and she wanted me to be the one who the fairy godmother made over and sent to the ball in really fancy clothes. I loved Cinderella because she knew that it was magic that made her fancy. It was not real. The real her was simple and more comfortable sitting in her quiet place watching everyone else have parties. I think that was how I was once the kids around me started hanging out and having parties. That happened around seventh grade. I was most familiar with my princess in hiding way of being, so I stuck with that. My sister Toni was the really big party girl. She was blond, athletic, outgoing, and popular. She had a lot of friends that were always over our house. I got to hang out with them because they were her friends, and they were always around. I was not really good at reaching out and making my own friends, so it was good to be able to have some adopted ones from time to time. Toni curled her hair and wore makeup. She also had some pimples and always put her makeup on in the dark. She said that she didn't want to see the pimples. I was lucky that way; I had no pimples and did not wear makeup. Cinderella would need no makeup or fancy hairdos to be a princess.

## 36 Shoo Fly Pie

"You are going to get fat eating all that Amish cooking!" Those were my mother's parting words to me when she dropped me off at Linden Hall. I was told that it was a privilege to go there and I was forced to attend. I am not clear why she these were her last words to me. Was she warning me or threatening me or convicting me to the imprisonment I was about to live? In one long breath she told me of the many dishes the cooks would prepare, full of butter and fat. One that stood out for me, because of its name was Shoofly Pie.[15]

The only food available to me was the fattening Amish food. And, I had was not allowed to skip meals. Attendance at every meal was mandatory as was the singing of Grace. However, the *Clean Plate Club* did not exist at Linden Hall. I had to sit at meals, but I did not have to clean my plate. I did not have to eat. So, I decided that I would not. I am not clear whether I did not want to get fat, did not want to follow my mother's command, or I just wanted to be in charge or something in my life. Anyway, most of the girls did get fat, or at least fatter. Even my cousin Sandy Dick Schwartz, who was a senior. I was fourteen and a freshman. There was only one other girl who did not eat at her meals. She was a senior and she was blond and beautiful, and her name was Nadine Bartomel She proudly announced to everyone that she would only eat when oysters were served. There were not a lot of oysters being served by the Amish in rural Pennsylvania, so Nadine mostly did not eat at mealtime. I found out later that she had a lot of snacks in her room. As for me, I was on a very strict schedule. I allowed myself one special food treat on Saturdays. There was a vending machine in the basement and from that machine I purchased my weekly ration of Walnettos, small chewy candies. Other than that, I did not eat but was never reprimanded for not being a member of the *Clean Plate Club*.

I did notice, after a while, that I was being watched. Like Nadine, people noticed that I was not eating, so, like Nadine, I got a lot of attention. It felt like good attention because people seemed to want to take care of me. There was a social system at Linden Hall called *Big Sisters*. Older girls, seniors, and juniors would choose a freshman girl to be their *little Sister*. *Big sisters* sort of took care of their chosen *little sister*, getting them special treats and giving them advise on just about everything. I never had a big sister at home as I was everyone's big sister, and the little mother, or as I called it, the Chosen Princess. I guess I never really had an older girl or a woman that wanted to take care of me. Here at Linden Hall, many, not just one, older girls wanted to be my Big Sister and take care of me. There were lots of rewards for not eating. And I did not taste even one morsel of Shoofly Pie.

## 37 Love Songs

We heard a lot of music as kids. There were only two kinds of songs, those that played on Mom's record player at home and those sung at the Presbyterian Church each Sunday. Home songs were *being in love* songs. Handsome men wearing suits with smooth hair and clean faces smiled on the record covers. They sang about being in love, about important jobs for ladies to do, about the right kinds of pretty clothes to wear.

Mostly, I think, the singers wanted grown-up ladies to stay at home, do the cooking and cleaning house jobs, take care of the kids, but never to look tired or sad when the dads came home. They also sang about how the most important thing in life for a woman was to have a man.

It was important that moms looked pretty and happy and dressed in party dresses whenever dads were around. We were lucky to have TV programs that showed us just how to look and act, especially if we were girls and wanted to grow up and be like our moms. Here are some of the shows: *Leave it to Beaver, Father Knows Best, I Dream of Jeanie, and Bewitched.* They all did a really good job showing us what we needed to know. Good boys had short haircuts and good girls had their hair in ponytails out of their faces. Everyone was always smiling, and the moms wore fancy dresses all day long. The only difference in the shows' parents and in-home moms and dads, was that TV parents never raised their voices while home parents often yelled at each other.

There was no yelling at church and that was why, I think, we all went there every Sunday. Mom got to sing songs in the choir, and when we were old enough, we got to sing in the junior choir. In church there was no yelling but there was also no talking except by the minister, Mr. Renton. We were only allowed to speak when the parts on the hymnals said "Congregation." Then we said something altogether after Mr. Renton said something. I didn't really understand what we were talking about, but I did like the quiet during church.

The songs did not make as much sense to me as did Mom's *being in love songs* did. Church songs were kind of like poems which had some words that made sense and others that did not. In some ways the songs were similar because they told us how to act so that we could be loved. I guess God was a man too because the songs always called him "he."

When I was in sixth grade, I started to hear new songs, mostly from a singing group from London called the Beatles. Everyone, even grownups, were talking about them. They looked different; they wore tight suits and had long hair. Their music, as far as I could see, was about being in love. But, in their songs, boys and girls both had the same kinds of jobs. The boys sang about being true to their girls. They got to be in love by just holding hands.

It seemed that in these songs there were no secrets. For example, Mom's home songs told ladies to pretend not to be angry or tired even though they were at the end of the day. They also told moms that the most important thing was how they looked. And the church songs seemed to tell us about pretend lives or those that we would get when we were dead. After I heard the Beatles sing, I wondered if God wanted to hold our hands or if we would have to wait until we were dead in heaven.

## 38 Listening

Every year elementary and high school students had to go to the school nurse for hearing tests. The tests took place in a little room, more like a little closet with a window in it. I sat in the little closet when I was in first grade, and all the grades after that. When I was in sixth grade, and at the middle school, I took a hearing test that made me confused. I didn't know which of the sounds were important for me to hear. For the test, when you heard a tone, you were told to raise your hand. I am not sure what about this was confusing. There were so many different kinds of sounds, and I was not sure which ones were important to listen to and show, by raising my hand, that I had heard it.

I thought that the nurse told me to listen for only one type of tone and then to raise my hand. As I was listening and hearing so many sounds, some loud, some soft, some quick, some that seemed to go one forever, I tried very hard to single out the special sound that I thought I should be listening for. I had misunderstood the nurse. She had meant for me to listen for *all* the sounds that were coming my way either alone sounds or many sounds happening at once. I wanted to do the right thing and to please her. I wanted to get a good mark on my hearing test. Because I was listening for just one tone that sounded the same every time I heard it, rather than to ALL sounds, I failed my hearing test. No one seemed to care that I failed except for me, and no one asked why I had just raised my hand for the one tone. And no one tried to fix my hearing.

When I was in sixth grade, I wondered why this hearing test seemed so different from the tests that I took in other years. It was only this year that I thought I should be shutting my ears to most of the sounds and responding to the important one. It had been easier when I was little; I just raised my hand for everything that I heard. In sixth grade, for some reason, I thought that I had to make choices as to the best sound to listen for. The only thing that I could think of was how familiar this test felt to me these days. Everyone was telling me something different about how to look and how to behave. My mom told me that I should look pretty all the time, and some of my friends' moms told me to just have fun and play. The people at the church had rules and mostly we were told that there had to be secrets. There were the people in our town that told me that I needed to have certain clothes and toys to be invited to their clubs and parties. My stepdad told me I should try to be a lawyer because *I would only need to sign my signature and make a thousand dollars.* Then there was the type of music I should listen to and the kinds of kids I should hang out with. Everyone was saying something different, and I was not sure which person or rule to listen to. I think that this was part of my confusion with the hearing test. I was old enough during the time of that test to know that I would need to make some choices and not to listen to everyone because all together, their voices sounded like a battlefield. I needed to figure out whose side I should be on, or if I should go and make my own rules like I had on the sixth-grade hearing test. I was always trying to do the right thing then, so maybe I was not ready for making my own rules.

## 39 Practical Jokes

When we were little and needed a lot of watching out for or nurturing, Mom was not a real presence. I was the big kid who did a lot of the watching out for and nurturing jobs. However, when we were older, and looking more like adults, Mom took on a new role. What we discovered, and what she shared with us then, was her humor. She was a great practical joker! She seemed to love engaging us in her jokes. We were there to watch the outcomes of her plans. This mom is the mom that I would miss when sent off to my fancy boarding school where I would learn to be a lady like the ladies we heard about in Mom's family.

Our house was right across the street from the town medical center. One of Mom's pranks was to have one of us call the office, in a disguised voice, and tell them that we were driving by and saw Dr. Sasky's car was on fire. We would then sit and watch out the window until Dr. Sasky came running out of the medical center front door, looking frantically for his car.

Another joke happened when a new family moved next door to us. They placed a large mailbox in front. Mom's joke was to have us take the mailbox and put it in another location. The next day the mailbox would show up at the police station. Daddy Tom was the local judge, and his office was there so we know about this from him. He did not know about our part in the mailbox caper. This prank went on for the whole summer with the mailbox being moved further and further away from their house. Eventually it ended up at one of the local beaches and stayed there without being claimed.

Another prank that comes to mind was the one that involved the local radio station, WLNG, that had a service like a talking Craig's List for offering things for sale. You could sell things on it. So, Mom had one of my brothers call and say that they were Mr. Dijon. He had a really fancy, maroon-colored Cadillac convertible and he always drove around in it with the top down. My brother, pretending to be Mr. Dijon, put the car for sale on the radio for a cheap price. Mom thought it was really funny that Mr Dijon was getting all these calls about the car.

I would not be allowed to do practical jokes at Linden Hall. I think that I really missed being naughty at home. Naughty was a lot more fun than was being proper. Being proper meant that I could not even talk to the local town people in Lititz, where the school was. Even though Mom went to Linden Hall, I think she was full of pranks even then. Practical jokes are done in private. Being a good girl is done to please the public. Which one would be the one to choose? Maybe Mom taught us that you had to be both.

## 40 Being Two

I am standing at the top of the staircase in my parents' house. I am two and this is what I remember about the house I lived in with my parents and my

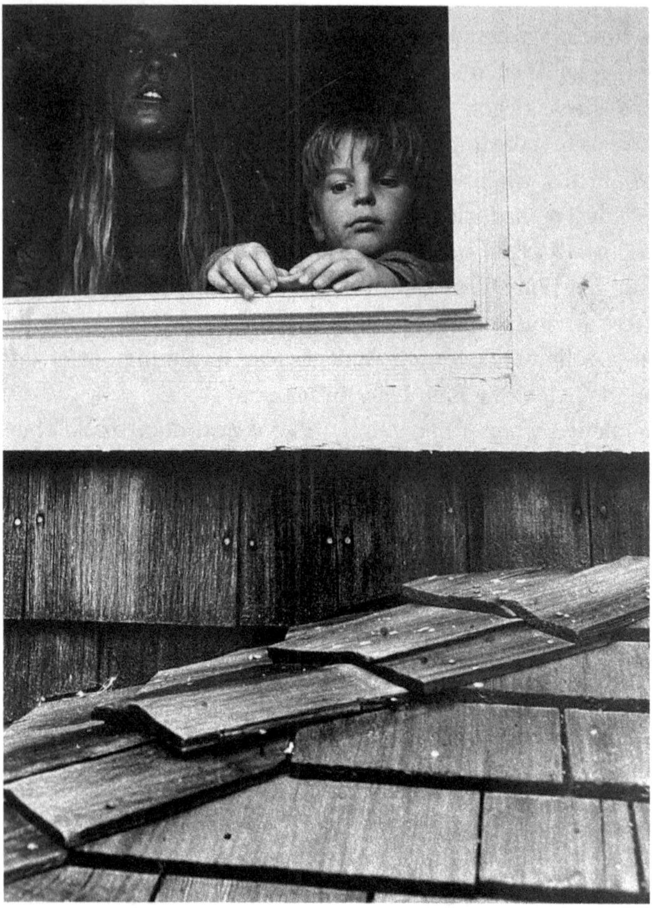

FIGURE 23 Prank observation tower: Pantigo Window, 1968

baby sister, Toni. She is one year old, and I am not happy to have her here with us. Mom does not hold me anymore because I am big, and Toni is a baby.[16] At the top of the stairs is a small chest from our bedroom. I think we share a bedroom. The chest is small and light enough for me to push from the room to the top of the staircase. The chest has four or five small drawers. I take one of the drawers out of the chest and put Toni in it. She is very small, like a baby, but I don't know how I was big enough to pick her up. I push her down the stairs in the drawer. It looks like a sliding board. I push her to the bottom and then my parents yelled at me. I think she was OK, but they are angry at me for trying to hurt the baby. This is the only thing that I remember about being in that house with my parents and Toni. Mom moved away from my father with Toni and me when I was two and a half. We moved to East Hampton then.

I do remember lots about Aunt Toni's house. Aunt Toni was my mom's much older sister. Mom named my sister Toni after her. I think that my aunt must have babysat Toni and me a lot while we were still living with her and my father. Maybe Mom had to go on trips while she was married to him. Anyway, even though I was only two, I remember Aunt Toni's house. It had a long hallway that led from the living room to the bedrooms. I stopped in that hallway a lot because there were lots of pictures hanging on the wall there. The whole inside of the house felt like it was green colored and there was a special basement. In the basement were lots of games that were set up for my cousin Ned. Ned was one year older than me. There was also a garage outside that looked like the garage at my grandparents' house. We must have spent a lot of time there because, later, someone told me that Aunt Toni weaned me from my bottle to a cup. I think that I must have not had much time nursing on my mom because Toni was born when I was one so she must have been pregnant while I was a baby.

I loved going to that house. Aunt Toni made lots of good food and always had hugs for us and read us stories. Her husband, Uncle Cass, was a funny uncle. Mom told me later that Uncle Cass had played golf with my father and that was how she, Mom, met my father. Mom loved Uncle Cass but always said bad things about golf. My father was a great golfer and started the golf club at Bucknell and had a score that was the same as a famous golfer, Sam Snead. All of that I found out later. I did not know about golf or Sam Snead when I was two.

## 41 Champagne Bubbles

Sunday was the day that we all got to watch TV together. The only TV was in my parents' bedroom and all seven of us kids lined up with pillows and blankets on the floor in front of their bed. It was a king-sized bed so there was enough room for all of us to lie down in a row facing the TV. There were three channels on the TV, and we usually watched ABC. I think that CBS was more of a news station and the other channel, NBC, was not one that we ever watched. "The Lawrence Welk Show" came on first. He was the host and had a funny accent and carried a baton. When the music played, he waved his baton and bubbles fell from the sky of the room. The bubbles kept falling throughout the show. There were a few acts on this show. One was the "Lennon Sisters" who were dressed in the same beautiful dresses, always with tight waists and full skirts. They had matching hairdos, which mostly were ponytails and bangs. They were always smiling and singing happy songs. I think they were happy songs because they were always smiling. Another act was a pair of dancers, Bobby and Barbara. Barbara wore dresses like the Lennon Sisters and Bobby always wore a suit. They also were always smiling and danced the polka. I know that because Lawrence Welk told us the name of their dances. Sometimes they danced to slower music, and it looked very romantic. I think this was a waltz dance. The other act that I remember was a beautiful older lady singer named Norma Zimmer. She always sang serious songs about God.

There were a few more shows that we watched together. In all of them the mothers wore dresses like the Lennon Sisters, but with aprons, and were always sending the children off to school and then, waiting for them to return. I think they must have been cleaning during the day and making dinner. Mostly, we didn't see them during the day. The fathers also were dressed like the men on the Lawrence Welk show. They wore suits and went off to work. Most of the half hour that each show was on was about the kids at school, getting into fun kinds of trouble, and being nervous that their parents might find out and get mad at them. They never did anything really bad. The names of these shows were: *Leave it to Beaver* and *Father Knows Best.*

During the time that we all watched TV at the bottom of my parents' bed on Sundays, I also found out about sex. I don't remember how, but I do know that I did not hear about it from my mother. I already knew about periods because she had already given me the Kotex book from 1945 to read. I guess this was in sixth grade. Maybe I heard about it from one of the older kids at school or read about it in a book that I was not supposed to read. I had not seen a picture of sex except in my imagination. So, one day I drew a picture of what I thought sex looked like. Somehow one of my parents found it. I know this because one day after school the minister from my church was sitting in the living room with my parents. They told me that they needed to talk about something serious. It was about my drawing. I was really in trouble. I am not sure why it was such a bad thing to make this drawing, but it must have been, because the minister was there to talk about it. I can't remember what they said, and I don't know what my punishment was. I do know that I was really embarrassed and hoped that no one else would know about this. Sex was a secret and was never talked about in school, at church, or on Lawrence Welk. I guess that all secrets must have been bad.

## 42 Invisible Rooms

My bedroom had two doors. My room, sitting between the two doors, became a runway for my six siblings. They were constantly running and chasing each other. My room was placed like an elbow, between two hallways. It was the only room in the house, other than the room downstairs with the record player, that had two doors. My room was not a nest. There was no place to be private. Maybe my closet was private. Only at bedtime did my room become quiet. Sometimes I would watch my brothers and sisters race through my room. They never slowed down. I felt invisible. They always seemed to be having fun. I don't know why I was not a part of the fun. For some reason, I always felt like I was on the outside of everything, watching. Even at the beach, where all kids hung out all day getting tans, I was different. I didn't like sitting still in the sun. I would go to the beach to swim. Swim and leave. I did not hang out with the other kids. I was the only one who stayed pale, even in the summer.

Mom always hung out with her friends and got too tan. I didn't like getting hot, but I did like the feeling of the sand, so I usually did not sit on a blanket, on a towel, or on a chair, at the beach. I wonder what everyone thought of me. I don't remember getting invited to join, either in the chase around the halls in my house, or with the sun-tanned kids at the beach.

I do know that my middle school art teacher thought about me. He wrote this in my yearbook: "To grade my friend Dicki gets a little bit sticky, because she and I know she tops. Her will and our effort climb and climb, till she's just about best- and then she stops." This poem made me think about how I never was best at anything.[17] He noticed that too but saw it as my choice. I guess not being part of the gang was my choice too. Maybe I wanted alone time because most of the time I had to take care of my younger sisters and brothers. I am confused because I know that I wanted to be part of the group but also wanted to be alone. Also, I think that I did not want to be the best. Mom wanted me to be the best so she could show me off. I just wanted to be like the others. I wanted to blend and to belong. I know that I tried dressing like my younger sisters so it would look like I was one of them even though we had different fathers and mine didn't live with us. I think that mom had wished that I had the same father as my sisters Ann and Robin. I know she told me to pretend that my last name was "Strom" and not "Johnson." There was a lot of pretending and of hiding some true stories. Maybe it was easier for me to hide behind the made-up stories if I was not the best. Being best meant that everyone was watching you.

## 43 Being Five

I already talked about my favorite birthday present from my fifth birthday. It was that beautiful blow-up slip. What I didn't tell was that I don't remember the party. I only remember that everyone had gone I don't know where everyone else was. Mom was probably with Ann, who was just one year old. I wonder why no one was around and what kind of birthday cake I had. Everyone else must have thought that I was practically a grownup because left me alone and you don't usually leave little kids alone. Maybe it was because I felt that this birthday was special because being *five* meant I was old enough to take care of myself. I don't remember any other birthdays except my *Sweet Sixteen*, which was much later. By the time that happened, I had a boyfriend who had

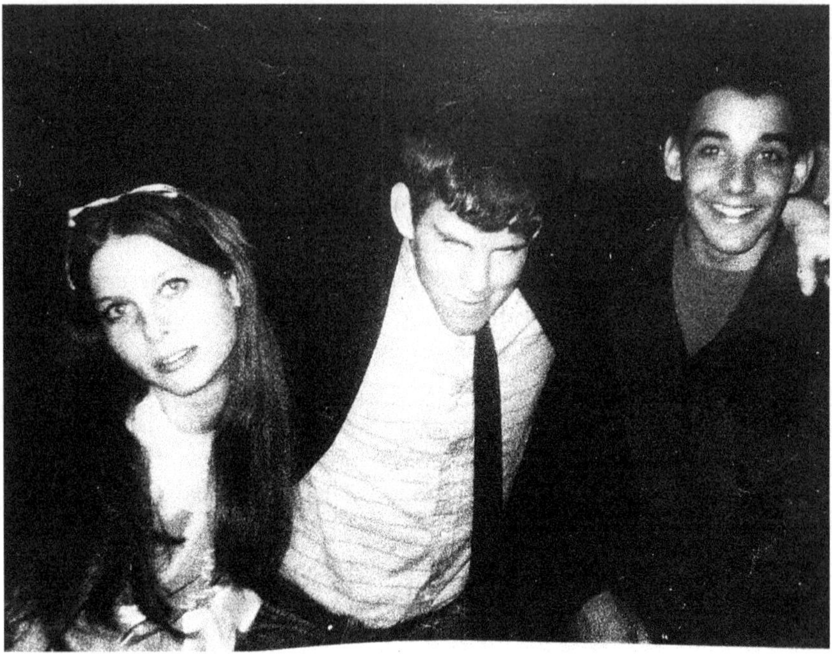

FIGURE 24 Sweet sixteen, 1968

a band called *The Zoo* and the band played at my party. I was dressed like *Alice in Wonderland* and the theme for the party was *Love is Blue*. That was the name of a song from my teens. I think that I felt more grown up at my five-year-old birthday than I did at my fancy Sweet Sixteen.

After I was five, mom had more babies. Tommy, Robin, and Randy came right away, one after the other and, since I was seven when they started to come, I was old enough to take care of them. Being five meant I was almost seven and getting ready to be junior Mom, or the princess of our house. Being five meant that I still wanted to be big, to be a pretty grown-up like Mom. Being five meant there was no reason to want to stay small. Five and six were good years. I lost my first tooth at my father's farm when I was six which meant I was on my way to being grown up with big-girl teeth. After that I don't remember birthdays, until my Sweet Sixteen. In between I must have been busy with other things. I can't remember when I decided it was better to be small.

## 44 Amish Tour Bus

It is very cold and dark. I am in a bus with the other Linden Hall girls. We are on an adventure. The adventure is not fun; there are no colors, no laughing, no songs. We are on a tour of Amish country. Our entertainment is watching the people do their chores. There are lots of cows and horses and wagons. The people wear dark clothes and cover their heads. The men have big farmer hats, and the women wear strange bonnets that look a bit like the head gear that nuns wear. There is a lot of outside activity with everyone working together, pulling wagons and buckets of water. We are told that they have no electricity and can have only buttons, no zippers, on their clothes. It feels to me like a foreign country, although I have never been to a foreign country so I imagine this is what it might be like. My cousin Barb told me that visiting my house was like going to a foreign country. It was crazy at my house; her house was calm.

Watching these people felt wrong. It reminded me of going to the zoo to watch caged animals. I never liked zoos because the animals looked so sad. I thought it was bad to take them away from their outside homes where they could run free. And the grown-ups at Linden Hall thought we would enjoy watching the strange Amish people who dressed so differently from us and did outside things we never did. Did they think it would make us appreciate having zippers and lights? Or was this just like going to the zoo to watch another kind of people? I did not know why we were there, but it made me feel sad and lonely. I was hungry and cold and wished that I could go and be outside with the Amish people and their animals. Instead, I was locked up in a bus looking out. I was like the animal that was taken from his home where he could laugh and run around with his family and friends. I was in the zoo. Were the Amish people looking us in that bus that looked like a cage and feeling sorry for us?

This thinking made me wonder about what it was like to die. Dying was an alone activity and I wondered if it was easier to die with animals and wagons and no electricity than locked up in a place like Linden Hall with no animals, lots of electricity, pretend smiles and fattening food which I could not eat. I just remembered that the Amish women made the food for the Linden Hall girls. Maybe if I ate their food, I could be more like them. All I knew for sure as I watched and asked myself these questions is that I was not sure which kind of girl I was supposed to be. I did know that if I got fat and wore Amish clothes my mom would not be happy with me. I really wanted to make her happy and be as popular and talented as she was. For now, I just had to work on being special, getting good grades and making her proud. I could do all of this and still not eat. That was what I could do for myself. It was a little confusing though. I felt strong because I was able to say "no" to all food and I was doing the Royal Canadian exercises that I found in some magazine and that made me special. But I was also feeling really weak because I had not eaten much at all for a few months, and I was really skinny. Maybe that is why I was feeling so dark and cold and thinking about what it was like to die alone.

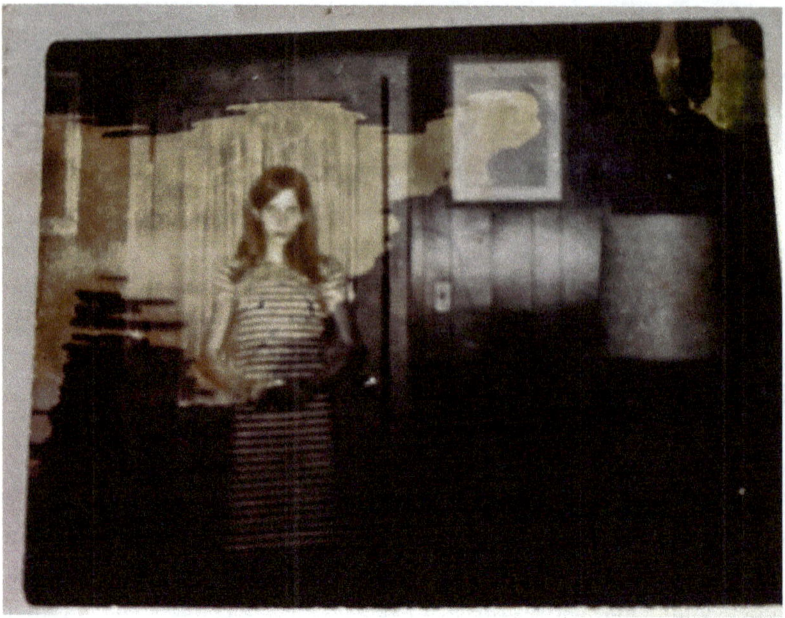

FIGURE 25 One month home, 1967

## 45 My Closet

My room at Linden Hall was not private. I had two roommates, Susan and Sally, and they were always in the room. If I got on the honor roll, I could study alone in my room at night when everyone else had to go to study hall. I got on the honor roll right away and got to have private time finally. I liked to look at myself in the mirror when no one was around and do my Royal Canadian exercises. Also, I would put half an "X" on the day on my calendar at the beginning of the day and the other half of the "X" at the end of the day. I didn't like to have my roommates watch me do that because they might think I was weird. I liked being alone although I got lonely when no one was around. That was a little confusing to me. I know that I missed the craziness of my brothers and sisters. Mostly I watched them run around and be crazy. Mostly, I was standing outside watching everyone. Here at Linden Hall, I could not be myself in my room when Susan and Sally were there because they wanted me to do things with them. I was different. They had their own way of doing things and they didn't understand that I saw things differently. They wanted me to eat snacks and I couldn't do that.

I missed my dog, Mitzi. She loved and understood me best. At school I thought that the headmaster was worried about me, so he gave me a special job to do every day. At the end of chapel, I was given a special brass snuffer and my job was to go to each pew, where there were tall candles, and put out the flames. It made me feel like an angel all alone in the chapel putting out the lights. I was not sure why I got this job as other girls didn't have special jobs. I thought that I looked like an angel with my small body. Maybe that is why I got that job, or maybe they were worried that if I was not happy, I would leave school and not finish at Linden Hall. While I was an angel putting out candles, I did feel happy. I was almost a Catholic.[18]

I went home for a holiday; I think it may have been in October. That was not a holiday for going home, but I got a special holiday because the school knew I really was feeling homesick. I'm not sure how I got home, but I think my parents picked me up because I remember thinking that I loved the long six-hour drive because I got them all to myself both ways. My mom made me her special German chocolate cake to take back to school with me. I put the whole cake in my closet in my room. It lasted two months, until I went home at Christmas. Sometimes on the day when I could have my Walnettos, I would take a small bite of the cake.

## 46 Pomeroy's Department Store

When Toni and I visited Daddy Bill, my father, in Berwick, he took us to buy fancy dresses at Pomeroy's. That was a really big store on the biggest Berwick street where all the stores were, and it was close to his new house. There was a bridge and a river close to that store. I think we drove over it to get to Berwick when he picked us up from East Hampton. His house was small, and we had to get to the front door by going down outside stairs. There was a soft chair in his room that he sat on and let us both sit on his lap together. I don't remember ever sitting on Mom's lap alone or with Toni. Next to his little yard was a fence that was for the neighbor's house. There were roses on the fence and when Daddy Bill was taking us to meet Mama Jean (she was not our stepmother yet), he picked two roses from that fence and gave them to us to give to her when we met her.

We didn't get to see my father a lot then. I think this story was when I was four and Toni was three. There is a picture of us together from this story. We are wearing the dresses that he got us at Pomeroy's. The dresses are yellow fluffy material with green velvet sashes. We picked them out ourselves, but Mom said they were tacky because she thought that Daddy Bill had picked them out. She never said nice things about him, so I am not sure why she let us wear the dresses for our Christmas picture. We have short bangs and haircuts. We look

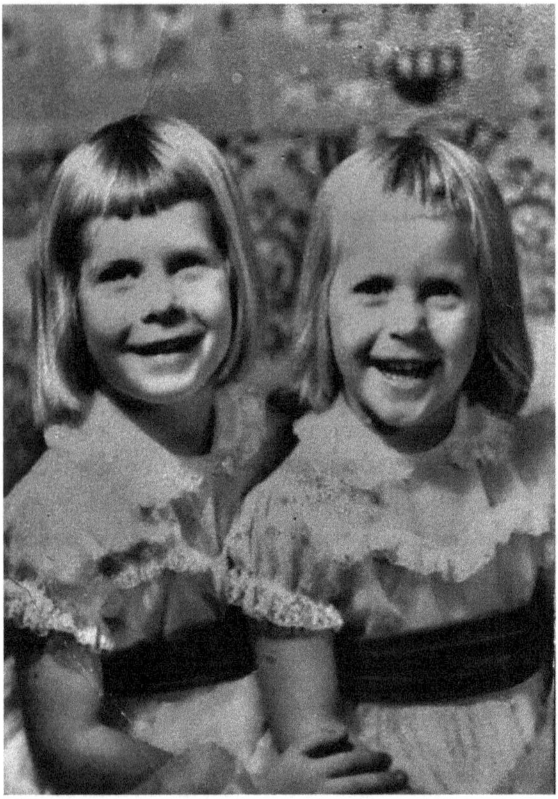

FIGURE 26 In daddy's dresses, 1956

happy and it looks like we are happy, and I think that is because we got to wear the dresses.

We are sitting on the couch in Mom's house on Church Street. This is the same couch we sat on for next year's Christmas picture with Ann, the new baby, sitting in the middle. Every year we had a new Christmas picture and mostly ever year, there was a new baby. I was always holding the new baby in the pictures. When there were three of us, Mom dressed us alike for the pictures but after that, we all had different outfits. Maybe she could not find clothes that were matched for so many children. I wonder what happened to my dress from Pomeroy's. I also wonder what happened to Pomeroy's because later it was gone, and Daddy couldn't buy us fancy dresses from there anymore. There was another store, Raccusin's, right next to his car dealership that had other kinds of clothes. When I was six, he bought me a sun suit with laces that tied on my shoulders.

I think we stopped dressing up so much after Mom married Daddy Tom and had so many more kids (except Easter when we all had Easter suits and hats and fancy shoes). There was always a picture of us in Easter suits although there were not any pictures of us in our regular clothes. We only got to wear those suits once because the next year we were too big for them. I wonder what happened to those Easter suits because I don't remember my smaller sisters wearing my pass-me-downs. Easter suits always had to be new just like babies always had to be new. Mom liked new babies better than grown-up kids.

I have come home for Thanksgiving after two months at Linden Hall. I am focusing in on an important job for this trip home. The job is coming up with the costumes for the kids to wear for the Christmas picture. I have decided that it is an important job. Mom used to think it was an important job, but she abandoned it after there were five of us kids to dress. I think maybe it was too hard to attend to us and to coordinate all those outfits. I must have learned that it was valuable from her when there were fewer of us, because every year, for our Christmas picture, we all had, either the same dress (when there were only girls) or color-coordinated dress clothes, when Tommy came on board. I, being the designated princess and coordinator of all things children, took over

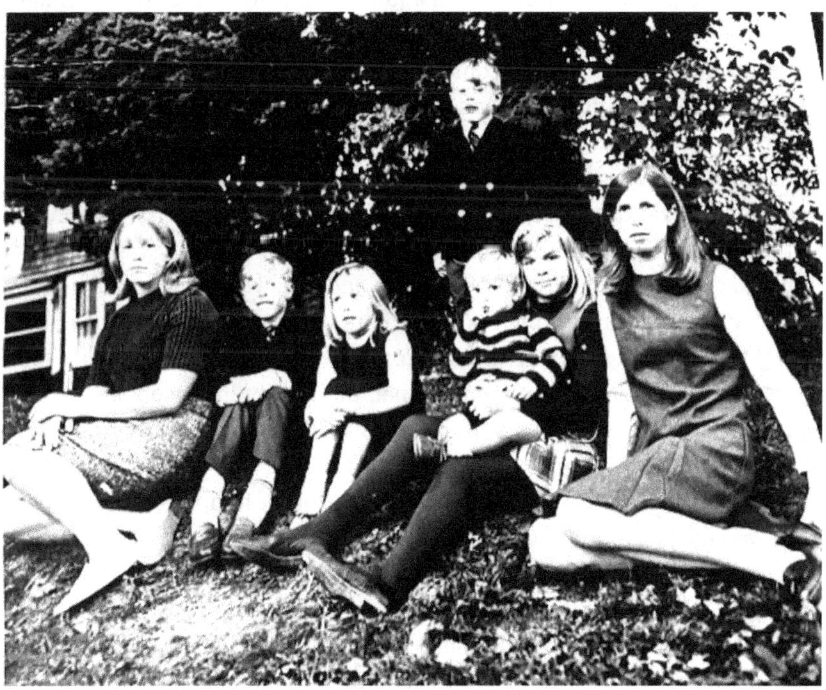

FIGURE 27 Color coordinated outfits, 1966

mom's abandoned role of dressing the kids alike. I think that in doing this, I am killing two birds with one stone. I wanted to please Mom and… if our clothes all blend with each other's, we would look like we belong to each other. I had so wanted to look like I belonged even though I felt otherwise. Remember, I have a different dad from most of my siblings. And remember, it made Mom ashamed for people to know that. She was ashamed that my dad was different. She didn't want people to think that she had taken too much; she always wanted everyone to see her as a victim or as a savior. That was confusing to me. I did know that she wanted me to pretend to be the same as her other children. That too was confusing because she made me different by sending me away to school. She wanted me to fit in but at the same time did not want that. I tried so hard to be one of them. Once I learned a little kid's song that was sung in German. Mom was always proud of being German and everything she associated with that background. The lyrics included counting to seven. There were seven of us children, so I taught the song to my sisters and brothers, and we sang it to my mom. It made me feel like part of a family.

When I came home, I began the task of finding outfits for us all for the Christmas picture photo shoot. As the boys always had navy blue blazers, I let that be the foundation color. I found a jumper in Ann's closet that was navy and maroon plaid with a blue top. I found a maroon sweater for her to wear under it. Ann, who will later become an angel, sits beside me and it is she that hold the baby, Billy. I have surrendered my crown to her. I have been carried away, on my mother's ancestral carpet, to keep alive the illusion of family legacy. In this foreign land of oceans, she was exiled to, she is determined to keep alive a family that has erased her. Three generations of women in her family attended Linden Hall. I guess I am chosen as sacrifice.

Toni had a dress that was maroon on top and tweed maroon on the bottom. The palette then became limited to these foundational two colors. Fortunately, I had a jumper that was a light maroon. Tommy and Randy each wore their navy blazers with navy and maroon striped ties. Baby Billy's wool little shorts outfit was navy and light blues stripes. Robin had a navy jumper with a light blue turtleneck under it. I also wore a turtleneck. Mine was pale yellow, which made me a bit different, color wise, but my combination of jumper with turtleneck under was almost identical to Robin's. She was my youngest, and smallest sister.

In the picture, I am sitting on one end of the lineup and Toni sits on the other. I am not holding the baby this time. In every other Christmas picture, I was tasked with holding the baby. I had become so thin that I was hoping to be mistaken for one of the younger of the children. In the photo, I am not sitting in my usual spot. Maybe I think that I am trying to trick everyone who looks at the picture into thinking that I am not the oldest. Toni, sitting on the end that used to be my spot, before I took over staging the photo, looks like the oldest. She is much bigger than me and even has a bit of a weight problem. She, however, is super popular and has lots of friends. She's the one who really knows how to be part of a group. She was never expected to be the princess.

### 47 The Red Chevy Belair

I am looking out of the living room window. This is our new house on Meadow Way that we moved into with Mom and our new Daddy Tom. Outside is a fancy red and white car with very big wheels. The wheels are mostly white, and the car is parked in front. I just remember it sitting there in front. I don't know what the inside looks like. Maybe Mom drives it with our new daddy and leaves us at home with a babysitter. I don't remember the babysitter's name only that I did not like having to stay with her while Mom went out.

The car must have come from my Daddy in Pennsylvania because he owned a place that sold cars. This was not a blue and white car like all of Mom's other cars so I think she must have gotten one of the cars that sat in Daddy's showroom. She would not have chosen a red car. It was very flashy. It looked like a spaceship with wings. I liked to look at it and wondered where we would go if Mom took us for a ride.

When we were living in the Meadow Way house, I was only three; I know this because we moved to Church Street when Mom had Ann and I was four then. I am mentioning my age because I think I must have been smart to notice all that I did about the car. I was smart but maybe not so nice because Toni got her mouth washed out with soap because of me. What happened was that the babysitter told me to do something that I didn't want to do so I told her to "shut up." In those days saying that was like a swear word. Also, in those days, if we said something bad, we had our mouths washed out with soap. That happened in school too, but not to me. Anyway, the babysitter was not really paying attention to us so when my mom came home the babysitter told her that one of us had said a swear. She could not remember which of us it was. I pointed to Toni and told Mom that she had said the swear. The thing is, Toni was only two, so she didn't talk much yet. She got the punishment instead of me. It is too bad when a person can't speak and defend themselves. It is also too bad that kids get left with babysitters who don't really pay attention to them enough to know the difference between two girls that look very different from one another. Those are the two things that I remember about being three and living in the Meadow Way house. One memory was outside, and one was inside: They were the red Chevy Belair and the mouth washed out with soap incident.

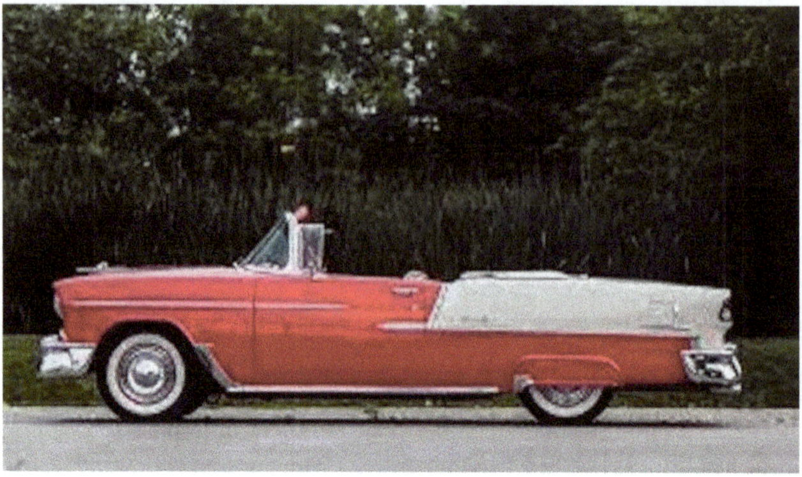

FIGURE 28 Chevy Belair, 1955

## 48 Mom, My Hero

Mom had warned me that if I ate the Amish cooking at Linden Hall, I would get fat. Or maybe it was not a warning but was her statement of fact, "You *will* get fat eating all the Amish cooking." She was in charge of me, and she told me what I would do. I think that she never asked me what I wanted to do or what I thought about what she had decided that I *would* do.

I simply decided not to eat. I don't think it was because I didn't want to get fat. At fourteen, I was not thinking about fat or thin. I was normal, I did not stand out as being special or different. Maybe as I got thinner, I became special and was noticed. I don't think that was behind it all. I do know that Mom was beautiful and thin and maybe I just wanted to be like her. She was my hero. If I got fat, I would not be like her.

At Linden Hall I took the following courses: Latin, Bible, Science, History and English. My extra courses, which I got to choose, were Voice lessons and English Riding lessons. Mom was a great singer and an equestrian and at her special school, I was training to be like her, so I took those electives. In English class, we had an assignment to write a paper about a hero in our lives. I wrote about Mom and how talented and wonderful she was. I think that this is important to know as I remember really believing that she was amazing and was a wonderful mother. I wanted to please her above all others. If I could be like her, maybe she would really love me. I don't think I really noticed what she didn't do for me until my siblings later pointed out her flaws especially that she neglected us.

As an older teenager, after I returned home to live, I thought about writing that hero paper and how odd it seemed to me then. I thought that I must have been seeing her through some kind of veil or fog. I was not seeing what might be under that veil. She *was* very special, but never let us, her children, get close to her. I don't think that I had a clue about what she really thought. She told us stories of her amazing growing up life, but they were her stories. Her stories were of glamorous past adventures, most of which took place at Linden Hall or at her college. After that, the stories seemed to end. Sometimes I wondered what happened next and how she met my father and got married. The stories were like dreams. For a while I wanted to have dreams and adventures like hers. The parts that I remember about our everyday life were different from her stories, so I got confused about what was real and how I should be. The easiest thing for me to do when I was fourteen was to copy her and to ford a path that mirrored her dream life. If I could be like her, maybe I could impress her. That seemed to be all I could do at that time. I do think that the *Mom* described in her stories was her favorite person. Even though I am not sure what parts of her stories were real, when I was fourteen, she was also *my* favorite person, my hero.[19]

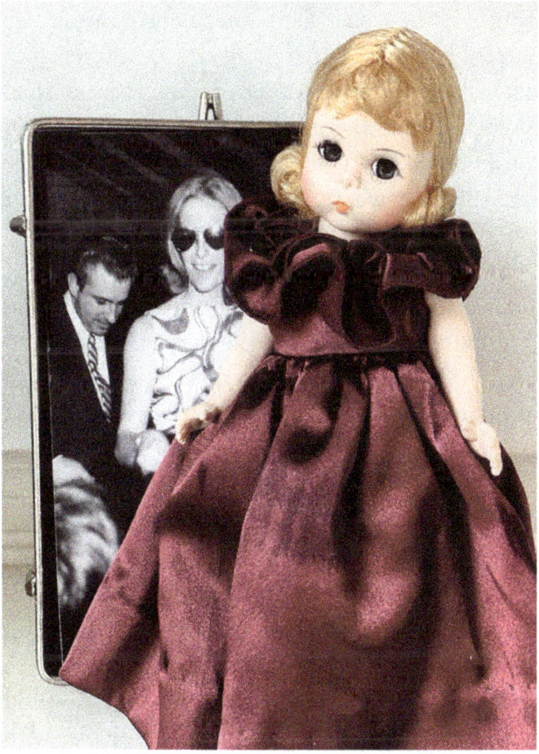

FIGURE 29 Mom and Red Madame Alexander Doll

## 49 The Untouchables

We were not allowed to touch some of Mom's special things. They were meant to be looked at or to be saved and passed down to us when our parents died. Most of these special things had been passed down to Mom when her parents died. On her dresser was a small, red leather round-shaped jewelry box. It had a zipper and inside were two layers of grey soft material. The top one had a few fancy jeweled pins attached to it. Under this layer were necklaces and a grey looped holder for rings. The most beautiful of the jewels was a pin with five rubies. I really wanted to wear that and hoped that I could get a chance before Mom died.

Mom talked a lot about all the things that we would get when she died like the wine glasses with the German cross on them. Mom said that they had belonged to her grandparents when they lived in Germany. They also had real gold on them, and my brother Tommy told me later that the cross looked like a Nazi cross. To me, at eight, the glasses just looked very pretty and expensive.

We were also not allowed to go into Mom's closet and try on her shoes. She had so many pairs of shoes! Her brother ran a fancy shoe place in New York City called Ferragamo. Mom told us that she had a very unusual shoe size because her feet were very narrow. She told us they were size AAA. Uncle Ned sent her big boxes of shoes in her size from Ferragamo. I imagined that she had princess-feet like Cinderella. When no one was around I would sneak into her closet and try some of them on. I figured that when I grew up, I would not have princess-sized feet so I might never get to wear them in real life. I would never be as pretty or special as my mom.

Something else that we were definitely not allowed to touch were the Madame Alexander porcelain dolls that Aunt Lois sent us for Christmases and birthdays. Madame Alexander dolls, Mom told us, were very expensive and came from FAO Swartz in the city. She kept the dolls in their blue boxes with pink tissue paper and she put them on shelves in our rooms. We were allowed to look at them but never to play with them.[20] I think that expensive things were meant to be loved for how they looked. We could touch and play with things that she didn't care about. It seemed she kept out of our reach possessions that reminded her of her parents and her rich aunts. She was always telling us how generous they were with their money. My grandparents died before I was ten but at eight, I had a few memoires of them in their big house with an elevator inside that was right across from the cemetery. They never came to visit us because they were old. My aunts sent us expensive gifts that we could not play with, but they never came to visit us. I wonder if Mom got to play with her expensive toys when she was little and if her family came to visit her? She

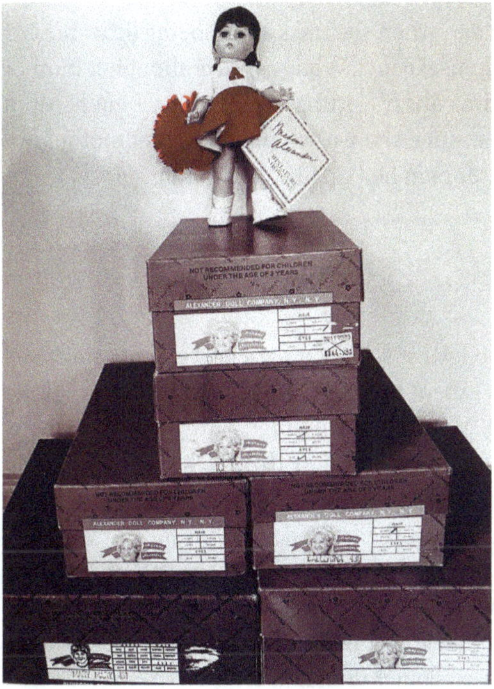


FIGURE 30
Red Cheerleader Pyramid, 2021

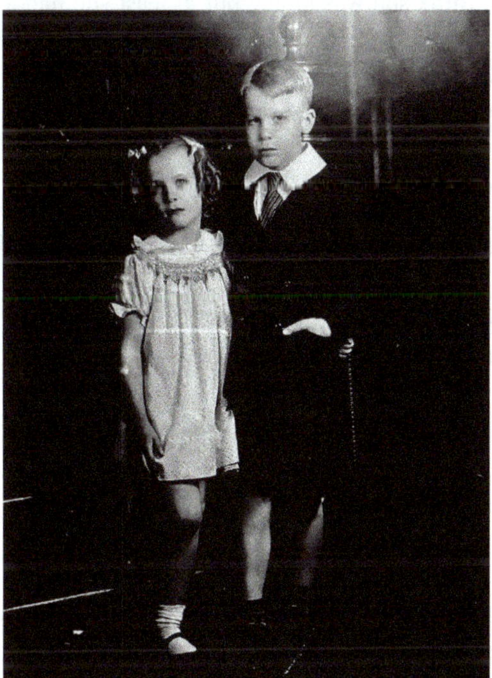

FIGURE 31
Portrait by Bachrach, 1934

was the youngest of ten children and when she talks about being little most of her stories were about Mary her housekeeper. What she says about her mother is that she was always old and was always sitting in her chair. I guess Mom didn't get to touch her too much, since she was so old. My grandmother, we called her *Bom-Bom*, didn't hold Mom in her lap like young moms do.

## 50 Photo by Bachrach

Two children are standing on the lowest step of a dark and gloomy staircase. Everything in the picture is dark except the little girl's smocked dress and the boy's starched collar. The photo, Mom always pointed out, was by a famous photographer, Bachrach. I wondered as a child, if this Bachrach was related to the Burt Bacharach that made all the songs Mom listened to when we were growing up. The two children are perfectly dressed, yet they looked very sad. Her arm is around his waist and his hand is in his pocket. This is a photograph of Mom and her brother Philip who died of a heart attack when he was in his 30's. He was the only sibling that she grew up with as all the other eight were between fifteen and twenty-five years older than her.

I wonder what it was like being the little girl with perfect banana curls who posed so well for photographs. I think she was lonely but at least she had a brother to play with. Maybe in those days girls and boys didn't play together. She did not talk about being little with us too much. She only talked about being a teenager with lots of boyfriends. I imagine that she didn't talk about being a little girl because it was not a happy time. There was a woman who was the mother of her best friend Marion, who told me that Mom always came over to their house because it was a warm and happy place to be. I think that Mom loved being there because Marion's mom cared for her in a way that Bom-Bom did not. I remember Bom-Bom's house feeling very dark and unfriendly. I don't think that Mom learned about being a mom from that place. I think that she looked everywhere for love. Maybe that is why she had so many boyfriends and only talked about that time in her young life.

It was important to Mom that we had our photographs taken by the same photographer in Pennsylvania. Mom wanted to please her parents and, I guess, did so in the only way that she knew how. Posing in matching clothes for portraits was what she did as a child and what she set up for her children to do each year. Most important was how we looked for those pictures. Most important when she was a child, was how she looked in pictures. Her older brothers and sisters were not in those photographs because they were adults when she and Uncle Phillip were children. When I was little, I thought when I was little, that

Mom wanted to have more children than Bom-Bom had. I am not sure why that was important, but, at least in the photographs, Mom had more and won the race. What was important, is how things looked, not how things really were.

### 51 Filet Mignon

I had two daddies. My East Hampton daddy was called *Daddy Tom* when we were in Pennsylvania. My Pennsylvania daddy was called *Daddy Bill* when we were in East Hampton. I called them both *Daddy* when I was with them. When we talked about the other daddy, he had a name that went with his daddy title. To make it clear, I will call the two daddies by their names when I talk about them here. Mom was never called *Mama Joan*, but my stepmother was always called *Mama Jean*, when we were with her and when we talked about her. Mom always told us in many ways that she was the *real* mom and that her kids were my *real* sisters and brothers. She was the queen of us all and made the rules.

When I went to Linden Hall, my mom would not allow my Daddy Bill to visit me at school even though it was in Pennsylvania and very close to his house. She said that he had not paid for the school, and she didn't want him to "parade around there looking like the big man." It was important to her that everyone at school knew that she was the one who had made the sacrifice and had paid for my tuition. This was too bad because I was very homesick at school. East Hampton was about six hours away so no one from home could come visit me. I really wanted to have my Daddy Bill visit me.

The story has other parts but this ending one is important. When I returned to Linden Hall after being home in East Hampton for Christmas, I didn't know what to do. In the term that ended before Christmas break, I had achieved all that was expected of me: I was the only freshman in all the clubs, I was the only freshman chosen to be a cheerleader and had the top-grade average not only in my class but in the whole school. There was nowhere from this point to go except down.

I continued my regime of exercise and starving, but I was not happy. I got sadder and also really thin; I was locked up in the school hospital. The doctors and nurses made me eat things that I didn't want to eat and would not let my classmates visit me. I was in lock-up until my parents came to pick me up and take me home. The school had decided that I was too much of a risk to keep in school. The decision (which I wanted all along I think) was made for me. The school was the bad guy, not me.

Mom was ashamed that I had not succeeded, so she did not come to pick me up. She would not look good to have a child that failed to keep her legacy going.

She sent Daddy Tom and my sister Ann to pack me up and bring me home. After we left Linden Hall, Daddy Tom took us to a fancy restaurant along the way home. I think that when I looked at the menu, I wanted to order the most expensive and luscious thing on the menu. I wanted to eat what I had not been able to eat at Linden Hall. The rules did not apply in the places between school and home. I ordered Filet Mignon.

## 52 Untouchables Part Two: The Plastic Runner

Mom's parents left her lots of money when they died. I was about seven when this happened. They also left her stocks in big companies like General Motors. She seemed proud to have those stocks. None of us kids understood about stocks, but they seemed like something that everyone would want. I am not sure what happened to all those stocks, but I do know that Mom was not great at managing money. When she had it, she bought lots of things and started going on trips with Daddy Tom and some of her friends. But there were times later when she didn't have all that money and made *Hamburger Helper* (that was a packaged meal she made for us) with eggs because she said she couldn't afford meat. I remember that right after she got all the money and stocks from her parents, she went on a couple of cruises to the Bahamas and St. Croix.

During that time, we also started visiting lots of big houses that were for sale. We were still living in the Church Street house smooshed into three bedrooms with two parents, six children and two dogs. It was lucky that she got all that money when it was time to get a bigger house. We didn't see the big Pantigo House before we moved into it. Mom spent a lot of time getting it ready and making it just right before we moved there. I think she wanted it to look like her, all blond and blue eyed. She always had cars that looked like her. They were light blue with white interiors. Looks were important to Mom: how she looked and how everything that was hers looked.

The living room looked just like Mom. It was covered in wall-to-wall light blue carpet, which went all the way upstairs on each stair. The couch was curved and big. It was big enough for all of us kids to sit on it. There was a problem: it was also light blue. This meant it could get dirty easily. The carpet had the same problem. Both looked really good in the Christmas pictures that we posed for. All the kids and the dogs were in those pictures. This living room was not a good place to play. Although most of the other rooms were not powder blue, they also had furniture and art things that were not good for touching or hanging out on.

Mom had a great plan for keeping her living room powder blue and clean. She did not want us messing it up, so she had a plastic runner put down on the floor that made a path up the stairs and through the room. It was like a little road for us all to walk on. We were not allowed to step off the plastic onto the blue carpet. She also put some of that plastic on the couch to protect it from us kids and from our dogs. Poor Mom, the plastic didn't work out well. Before long we were running off the path and jumping on the couch. I think she gave up trying to keep the house looking like her. She gave up when things didn't go right for her. I think it was the same with having babies. She liked them before they could talk back so maybe she just gave up and moved on to the next baby. This is what I though even when I was a kid.

There were too many of us to keep off the carpet and we just wanted to have fun. It was fun at first to try to walk on the plastic, but that kind of fun didn't last for long. Later on, I think we won because the carpet was gone, and my brothers put a ping pong table in the living room. It took up most of the room and all of our friends liked to hang out at our house when Mom stopped having rules and plastic runners.

## 53 Lots of Handsome Doctors

There were lots of doctors in our lives. It seemed to me that we all had earaches or hearing problems at the same time, or trouble with our bones, or stomach problems. Mom would pack us all in the car and take us to the doctor that was in charge of fixing what was wrong with us all at the time. It was strange that we all had the same problems and that we had to go back over and over again to the doctor. Mom seemed to like going to the doctors' offices. I am not sure that we were really sick. Maybe she just liked being around the doctors. Then, I was ten, Toni was nine, Ann was six, Tommy was four, Robin was three and Randy was two. Billy had not yet been born. We really didn't question what Mom did with us because she was our mother and we thought that she knew everything.

Later, when I was fourteen and had returned home from Linden Hall. I was taken, this time on my own, because I was the only one that had stopped eating and was really skinny, to one of her favorite doctors. I was thinking then that all of her doctors were very handsome. I was thinking that she has collected doctors in her grownup life, like she had collected handsome boyfriends when she was a teenager. Maybe that was not true, but it was an idea that I had when she took me to the doctor that time.

The doctor was handsome, but I thought he might not be very smart about girls who stop eating. Remember, no one asked me why I had done this. No one suggested that I might talk to someone about what I was thinking or feeling. The doctor just decided that the goal was to make me gain weight. And I thought, "No way am I going to do that." He gave me some pills to take and some powder to put in milk to drink. Both, he assured Mom, would fatten me up. The problem was, as I saw it, I was smarter than they were. I would empty the fattening stuff out of the pills (they were gel caps which opened in the middle) and just swallow the empty capsules. And, when no one was looking, I flushed the powder down the toilet.[21]

I guess that back in the 1960s doctors didn't think that feelings had anything to do with being sick or not eating. Back then doctors and parents had rules that they made us follow and one of the rules had to do with eating and not being skinny. I think that not eating was the only way that I could be in control and shape my body to look the way I wanted it to look. And besides, people really took care of me when I was skinny. At Linden Hall and even when I returned to East Hampton High, older girls seemed to rally around me in a special way. Before I was just average, and no one really took notice of me. I was not going to give that up, even though I am not sure why I stopped eating at the beginning. I remember that Mom said I would get fat by eating the Amish cooking and maybe, for once, I wanted to prove her wrong. Or maybe I just wanted to go back home and live with my sisters and brothers and all the animals.

I do remember that I did everything at Linden Hall that Mom expected me to do, but I was not happy. It was a dark and lonely place with too many rules. Especially awful a rule was the one where Linden Hall girls were not allowed to talk to the locals. I was pretty upset by that and confused about how, when I lived at home, I was not really a local and not really a country club girl. I guess the country club people looked down on the locals and I didn't know which group I should belong to. Being skinny I realized when I returned to East Hampton, also made me look like a model. Twiggy was the hot model at the time. I had not been aware of the fashion shift when I was at Linden Hall because it was a Moravian Church school and we had to be super dressed up all the time.

Now at home with a doctor trying to make me fat, I thought that he was stupid and was not sure if it was his idea or Mom's to force me to eat and take weight gaining medicine.

## 54 Daddy's Lap

Kids need hugs and need to have time on their parents' laps.[22] I know this is important because of something that happened to my little sister Robin. I don't' remember getting hugs or sitting on laps, but there was a photo of Toni

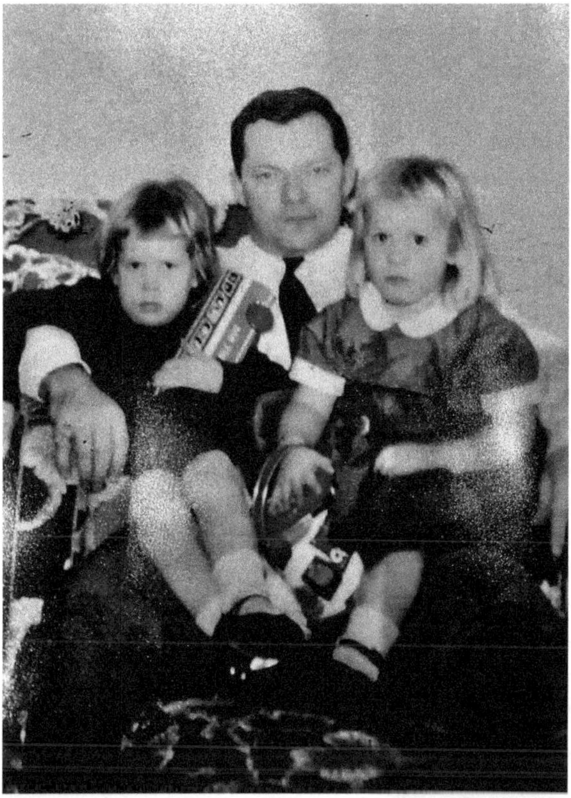

FIGURE 32 On daddy's lap, 1956

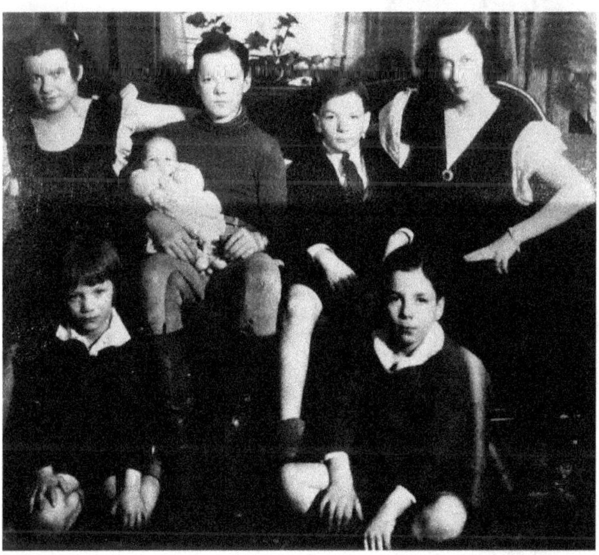

FIGURE 33 Baby on daddy's lap and other siblings, 1935

and me sitting on Daddy Bill's lap at his new house after Mom took us away from him to live in East Hampton. So, I know there were at least some lap sittings for me.

Robin is my sister from Daddy Tom. She was number five in the line of the seven of us. When she was about two and I was nine, she got bald in the back of her head. All the hair just fell out for no reason. Mom took her to the doctor across the street and he told her that what Robin needed was to be hugged. I thought that this was really cool. All she needed was some love just for her. This same doctor, five years later, was very different with me. I think maybe all I needed was some hugs and love rather than pills to make me fat. I wondered why this doctor didn't think of that.

Mom brought Robin home, but I don't think that she hugged her. She probably didn't have time to sit quietly with her. Like I said before, she was good at being patient with Parley, her horse, but not with us kids. I don't think it was her fault; it was just that no one taught her how to sit and hold kids. She was the youngest of ten children, didn't get to practice holding little brothers and sisters, and I don't think her mom held her. Maybe her dad did because she has nicer things to say about him.

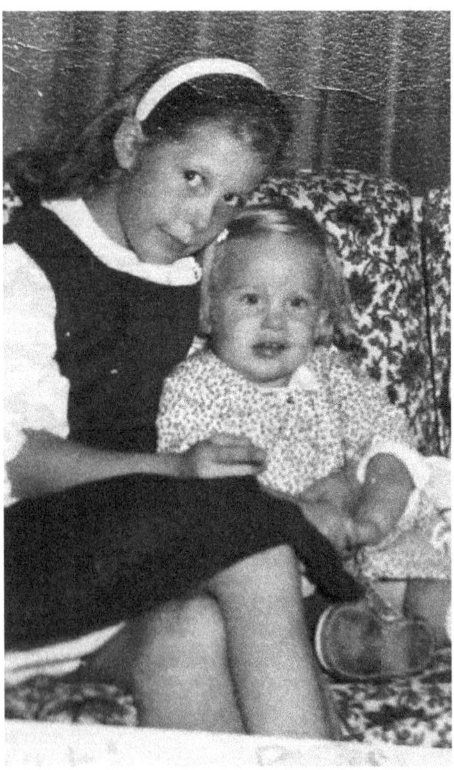

FIGURE 34
Baby Robin on Dicki's lap, 1960

Daddy Tom was the one that had the time to hold Robin. Even though he was the town judge and worked all day, he still made time every day to sit and hold her for a long time, in his lap. He was as quiet and kind with her as Mom was with Parley and Mitzi was with me. He would sit with her in her little room. There was no talking, just holding. What happened next was really a miracle. I don't remember how long it took but slowly her hair grew back. No one really talked about it or made a big deal of it. Maybe this was because Daddy Tom did not make a big deal of it. I don't think he was trying to get attention for being a good guy because he sat with her in private. It was OK for us to see him, but he did not ask us to do so. Maybe if he wanted attention, he would have sat with her in the living room where everybody hung out. I think he just wanted Robin to have his alone attention. I guess he believed what the doctor had suggested. After her hair grew back it never fell out again.

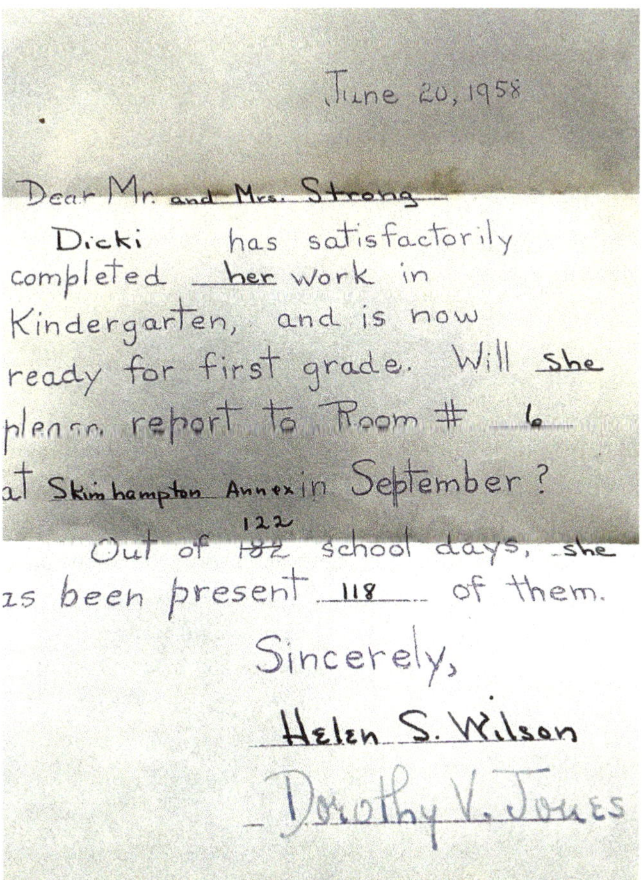

June 20, 1958

Dear Mr. and Mrs. Strong

Dicki has satisfactorily completed her work in Kindergarten, and is now ready for first grade. Will she please report to Room # 6 at Skimhampton Annex in September?

Out of ~~182~~ 122 school days, she as been present 118 of them.

Sincerely,

Helen S. Wilson

Dorothy V. Jones

FIGURE 35 Promotion notice, 1958

## 55 All Alone on the Prairie, My Horse and Me

There is only one song that I remember learning in First Grade. I was six and I learned the song by heart and could remember it and sing it forever. First grade has a lot of songs but I only remember this one so it must be important to me. Here is how it goes:

> Oh I wish I was a cowboy
> on the ranch all day long
> just a riding and singing
> a cowboy song.
> Got a trusty old pony
> and a pair of new boots
> I'm a wearing my six guns
> that really shoot.
> So get along get along get along
> it's time to go
> I'm headed to Texas for the rodeo.
> and if I was a cowboy
> oh how happy I'd be
> all alone on the Prairie
> my horse and me.

This song reminds me of Mom and her horse Parley. Parley was her horse and only she could handle him or ride him. I think that Parley came to her from a bad person who beat him. Whenever anyone got close to him, he would put his ears back. That meant that he was angry and might bite you. He didn't put his ears back when Mom was around him. She moved so slowly when near him and stroked his mane and he seemed calm. Around her, he was like another horse. Mom was proud that she was the only one who could handle Parley. He was very smart and could untie the knot on the rope that held his gate closed. Sometimes he got out of the corral and went into town and just hung out there where all the stores and people were. The police knew our family well because Daddy Tom was the town judge so maybe they let us get away with things. We were not really allowed to have horses if we lived in East Hampton Village, and we did. So, the police would call up Mom and say, "Joan come get your horse." It was funny because a horse is so big and the way they made it sound was like she should come pick up her dog that had gotten loose.

Mom was patient and kind with animals. I think that she passed on to me the gene for being more comfortable with animals than with people. I was thinking about how my dog Mitzi was my best friend. She waited for me every day while I was in school. She was patient with me like Mom was with Parley. I'm not sure where Mom learned about being patient with animals. I know that she rode horses at Linden Hall, but I am not sure what animals she had when she was little. I think that she had a dog because I remember a photo of her with a dog.

I liked watching her with Parley. I sometimes wished that she spent quiet time with me like that. But I had Mitzi and when I went to Linden Hall and was really lonely, all I wanted to do was talk to Mitzi. I was allowed to call home once a week on Sundays and I always asked my parents to put Mitzi up to the phone so I could talk to her. I knew that she was listening to me because she loved me, and I loved her.

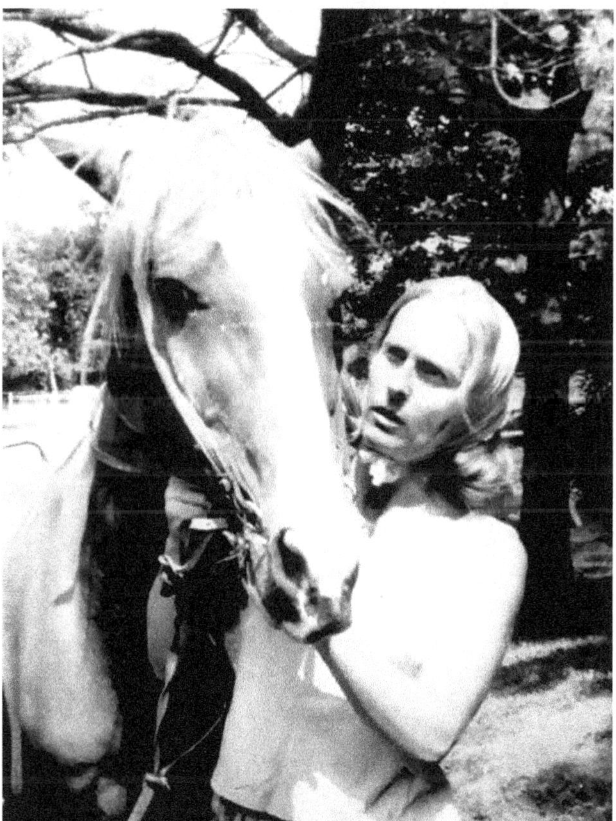

FIGURE 36 Mom and her Horse Parley, 1965

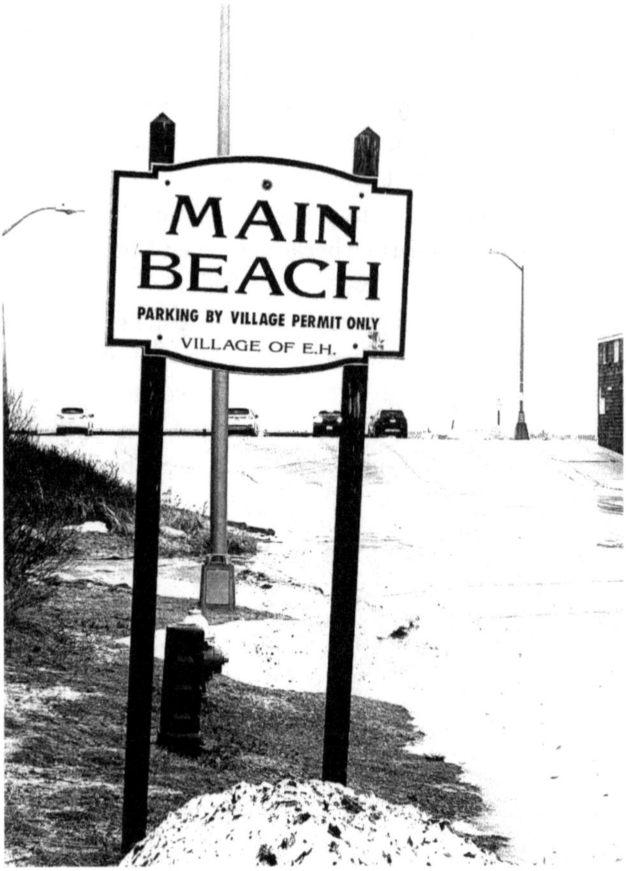
MAIN
BEACH
PARKING BY VILLAGE PERMIT ONLY
VILLAGE OF E.H.

FIGURE 37 Main beach parking lot

## 56 Bitten

I cannot believe that I am with Casey. I am smitten. I am in eighth grade, and he has invited me to Main Beach with his crew to ride skateboards in the parking lot. Facing the beach, the parking lot is steep; at the top, we can look out on Main beach. I have so many memories from being little on this beach. It was our first outdoor playground when we landed here with Mom after we left Pennsylvania. Most of the time we were on the beach, playing in the sand or running into the ocean and diving into waves if the flag was white. There were three types of waves, and each had a flag color to tell everyone, especially moms and kids, if the waves were safe. White flag meant it was calm, blue flag was medium rough and red flag meant the water was dangerous with undertows. If there was no flag, a hurricane was coming.

Today I can see the beach and the waves, and it feels like I am on top of a mountain. I feel like I could fly over the ocean. I stand on Casey's skateboard in front of him and he holds my waist. Being close to a boy is new for me and I want to stay here on the skateboard forever. It is as if I am looking out on the stage of my childhood and getting ready to become a teenager in love. Freedom in this moment. I am looking down on the world rather than up at all the grownups who tell me what to do. I am free from all those different voices and all I hear is one voice, the voice of my heart.

Mom is wanting me to go to Linden Hall for ninth grade, which is next year. I don't think that I want to go there but she says that it will be a good experience for me. I have looked over the brochure many times trying to get a feel for it. But I can't think about that now because I am on Casey's skateboard, and he is holding onto me which means that I am his girlfriend. Before laying eyes on him I didn't think I would want to have a boyfriend. I saw him first when he came to our house to take Toni on a date. He is skinny with round glasses and not her type. She likes football players. And somehow, I got to be with him. I am not sure how that happened. I just wanted it to be so. Sometimes when you really want something to happen, it does. He smelled like English leather. That was a perfume that boys wore back then.

For sure liking Casey was not going to be enough reason for Mom to let me stay at East Hampton High School for ninth grade. There were other plans for me. What I do know is that when I came back to E.H.H.S. I was very skinny from not eating and Casey didn't want to be my boyfriend anymore. Someone told me that he said about me: "I can put my arm around her and put my hand in my pocket."

Maybe boys want fatter sexy girls and so boys don't pay attention to me when I am skinny. I am not sure who I want to pay attention to me. I know that older girls want to take care of me, and I like that because I never had an older sister. I do feel sad that Casey doesn't want to be my boyfriend in ninth grade. I do remember that I made a *Casey Box* that had lots of things in it that reminded me of him. I carried it everywhere with me because it made me feel like he was with me. I could hug it and hold it close to my thin body. Really, he didn't think of me at all.[23] I did not want to get fat, but I wished that I could be glamourous and sexy without being fat and blond. I have become like one of Mom's untouchable possessions. I am finding myself to be like those Madame Alexander dolls that are left in their boxes to look at and not be played with.

When I returned home from boarding school, I noticed that my skinny body looked like the models in the magazines. I was becoming the image everyone likes to look at but not touch. I was not planning on this when I stopped eating at Linden Hall. Now more than ever, no one cared about what I thought, but now, at least, I was getting attention for how I looked. I was in charge of my body even if no one wanted to hold it. I can't think about that now. Maybe tomorrow.

### Notes

1 Snapshot. (n.d.). Definitions.net. Retrieved February 4, 2022, from https://www.definitions.net/definition/snapshot

2 The snapshot concept was introduced to the public at large by *Eastman Kodak,* which introduced the Brownie box camera in 1900. Kodak encouraged families to use the Brownie to capture moments in time and to shoot photos without being concerned with producing perfect images.
Snapshot (photography). Wikipedia.com

3 Theme: Excessive collecting as result of anxious attachment for child of inconsistent mother: "An anxious attachment style is associated with a tendency to anthropomorphize comforting objects and an inability to tolerate distress, which in turn leads to excessive acquisition" (Norberg et al., 2018).

4 "For girls initiation begins with the appearance of the first menstrual blood. This psychological symptom the sign of sexual maturity compels a break… the young girl's removal from her familiar world… the sacred ground her physical isolation symbolically separated from the conditions of her earlier life from the mother and from her childhood" (Chernin, p. 170).

5 There is a tendency to dissociate when feeling out of control, especially when forced to follow that are restrictive.

6 The beginning of being silenced. "It is my aim to fight back against the tendency to silence anorexic women's criticism of their treatment and the way in which they are described in public media, and to underline the need to listen to anorexic women views of the discourses and practices that are allegedly helping them" (Saukko, 2008, p. 34).

7 "Women today because they cannot bring their natural body into culture without shame and apology, are driven to attack and destroy that body. We have followed the tendency as aggressive position against the female body in psychological terms drawing it out from the original mother child relationship" (Chernin, p. 186).

8 Theme: Pretense of belonging to be accepted into social groups.

9 *Dressage* (/ˈdrɛsɑːʒ/ or /drɪˈsɑːʒ/; a French term, most commonly translated to mean "training") is a form of riding performed in exhibition and competition, as well as an art sometimes pursued solely for the sake of mastery. As an equestrian sport defined by the International Equestrian Federation, dressage is described as "the highest expression of horse training" where "horse and rider are expected to perform from memory a series of predetermined movements" (https://en.wikipedia.org/wiki/Dressage#cite_note-1).

10 Theme: Pretense of belonging to be accepted into social groups. False persona in lieu of true expression of self.

11 Theme: Mother's frustrated dreams:
"Bruch argued that the problem was that anorexic mothers, women of superior intelligence and education, was that they had given up promising careers or other ambitions in favor of family and children. This only left them unsatisfied. Neurotically focused on their children

they were trying to inculcate them and especially the anorexic daughters to live up to their own frustrated dreams" (Saukko, 2009, p. 52).

12 Theme: Ambivalence toward mother:
"The ambivalent child seems to be desperately trying to influence her mother. Many of them seem *hooked by her haphazard, unpredictable style* and the fact that she does come through on occasion. They pick up that she will respond sometimes, perhaps out of guilt, if they plead and make a big enough fuss" (Karen, 1998, p. 221).

13 Hilda Bruch (1978) argued that anorexia is caused by a "paralyzing underlying sense of ineffectiveness" (p. x). they have eaten the food that has been put on their plate without complaint, they have achieved high grades at school without really considering their goals, and pursued careers that they have not chosen. Anorexia is the final rebellion of these women who have never before caused any trouble" (Saukko, 2008, p. 27).

14 Theme: Lack of cultural rituals for transition into woman hood.

15 Shoofly Pie
- For the crust:
- 1 1/4 cup (175 g) all-purpose flour
- 1/2 teaspoon kosher salt
- 1/2 teaspoon white sugar
- 1/2 cup (115 g) cold unsalted butter, cut into 1/2-inch cubes
- 3 to 4 tablespoons water
- For the crumb topping:
- 1 1/2 cups (210 g) all-purpose flour
- 1/2 cup (110 g) packed dark brown sugar
- 1 teaspoon ground cinnamon
- 1/2 teaspoon ground nutmeg
- 1/4 teaspoon kosher salt
- 1/2 cup (115 g) cold unsalted butter, cut into 1/2-inch cubes
- For the filling:
- 3/4 cup (230 g) molasses, light or regular strength
- 3/4 cup (160 g) hot water (from the tap is fine)
- 1/2 teaspoon baking soda

The unusual name of shoofly pie came from "the fact that pools of sweet, sticky molasses sometimes formed on the surface of the pie while it was cooling, inevitably attracting flies." She suggests the pie's invention stems from Pennsylvania Dutch farm wives making do with what remained in the larder during the late winter. (Bird-in-Hand.com)

16 "The avoidant child is very controlled, and his anger more likely to be cruel and bullying, a reflection of an underlying hostility that has been redirected towards a safer target" Karen, R. (1998). *Becoming attached: First relationships and how they shape our capacity to love.*

17 Example of evolving Imposter Syndrome wherein one internalizes belief systems which lead to self-doubt.

18 Theme: Connection between self-denial, spirituality and purity: "The decoding of slenderness to reveal deep associations with autonomy, will, discipline, conquest of desire, enhance spirituality, and purity, and transcendence of the female body suggests that the continuity's proposed by Rudolf Bell between contemporary anorexia and the self-starvation of medieval Saints are not so far-fetched" (Bordo, 2009, p. 69).

19 "This is the hunger knot in which identity, the mother separation struggle, love, rage, food and the female body are all entangled. We must unravel patiently meticulously strand by strand until we know ourselves" (Chernin, 1985, p. xiv).

20 Mom, as a grandmother, bought countless porcelain dolls for my daughters to play with. The problem was that she did not do so until they were grown women. As a grown woman, I recently purchased seven vintage 1960s Madame Alexander dolls. I am not sure why, but I felt a sense of empowerment in being able to take them out of the boxes and hold them. I will save them for my grandchildren and encourage them to play with them. Attached to each doll is a flyer from the company which suggests that children should enjoy playing with the doll.

21 "Behavior modification was especially popular in the 1970s, although it is still often used in combination with other therapies. The anorexic is rewarded with positive reinforcements when she eats and negative reinforcements when she refuses to eat. If the patient doesn't eat she can be tube fed, isolated, or ordered to bed rest" (Saukko, p. 19).

22 Virginia Satir, world-renowned family therapist had advised: "We need 4 hugs a day for survival. We need 8 hugs a day for maintenance. We need 12 hugs a day for growth" (Satir, V. 2011, Jan 18). Magic touch: Six things you can do to connect in a disconnected world. *Forbes.*

23 My focus upon pleasing Mom seems to have been transferred to my obsession with Casey, my first romance and later to others as well as to female teachers. "They [ambivalent children who become anorexic] are wildly addicted to her [mother]and to their efforts to make her change, they become enmeshed with her in various unhealthy ways, and later in life they become similarly addicted to other potential attachment figures, such as teachers in the school years and, in all probability romantic figures after that. But through it all they do not believe they have what it takes to get what they need from another person" Karen, R. (1998). *Becoming attached: First relationships and how they shape our capacity to love.* New York. Oxford University Press (p. 222).

# PART 2

## *They Speak*

CHAPTER 2

# Let's Start at the Very Beginning...

## *Safety, Trust, and Attachment*

> Dance along with song originates in the leaping and wailing of infants.
>
> PLATO, LAWS (816a)

∵

## 1 Introduction

How we are launched predicts, or at least influences, who we will become and the types of relationships we will develop. An infant's initial relationship with her primary caregiver sets the stage for this launching. The developmental term for this relationship is *Attachment.*

Attachment Theory is based upon the combined visionary experiences of Mary Ainsworth and John Bowlby. The developmental history began "with Bowlby's growing interest in the link between maternal loss or deprivation and later personality development and with Ainsworth's interest in security theory" (Bretherton, 1992). Developmental theorists, psychologists and physicians agree that maternal relationships that are sustained, consistent, and responsive lay the foundation for security in the child's sense of self. The following equation reflects the impact which dynamic relational styles may have upon emotional launching:

> Sensitive Mother = Secure Child
> Inconsistent Mother = Ambivalent Child
> Interfering Mother = Avoidant Child

Erik Erikson (1950) states: "The amount of trust derived from earliest infantile experiences depends on the quality of the maternal relationship" (p. 249). Children seek consistency when listening and looking for safety.

The lack of secure attachment may position girls to later adapt destructive social coping mechanisms. Adaptations, in the service of survival, develop when there is an absence of external (parental, societal, global) support or

 | DOI:10.1163/9789004711051_003

safety. Current research continues to explore the relationship between initial attachment and the development of Anorexia:

> Considering the multifactorial nature of Anorexia Nervosa, the important place of the family and the growing interest in the Theory of Attachment in eating disorders, parental bonding is questioned in Anorexia Nervosa. (Albinhac, 2019, p. 121)

## 2 Neurobiology and Prenatal Influence

Porges' (2011) research in neurobiology tells us:" Specific areas of the brain detect and evaluate features, such as body and face movements and vocalizations that contribute to an impression of safety or trustworthiness" (p. 13). The child looks, listens, and feels for safety in the world around her, and initially, her mother is that world. Success in finding this safety jump starts her toward healthy identity development:

> The earliest verbal, tactile, and auditory interactions between the mother and infant actually helped determine the growth and chemical structure of the brain, leading to the development of personality characteristics and ultimately the person's sense of self. (Scaer, 2007, p. 131)

Consider what happens when the bodies and faces in a child's social and physical environments, communicate contradictory messages. The child appraises this chaotic environment in search of someone or something familiar. The familiarity means safety to her. After a while however, there may be many familiar and consistent people in her world. If the many disagree with each other and tell her different stories, how will she appraise which is the story she can trust.?

> A child's nervous system may detect danger or a threat to life when the child enters a new environment or meets a strange person. Cognitively, there's no reason for them to be frightened. But often even if they understand this, their bodies betray them… This explains why a baby coos at a familiar caregiver but cries at the approach of a stranger, or why a toddler enjoys the parent's gentle embrace but interprets the same gesture from a stranger as an assault. (Porges, p. 12)

Odent (1999) investigates the impact which the child's prenatal environment and the subsequent birth process have upon identity development. He suggests that the type of birth process that one experiences has long-term social consequences upon both one's ability to love and their proclivity toward aggressive. This association interests me as I consider the impact which my birth process had upon my identity development. Mine was a difficult birth. I was pulled from my mother's womb with forceps and was, initially, unable to breathe. With my first breath, I experienced the world as controlling. I was not allowed to bring my body into the world naturally, rhythmically attuned to the waves of my mother's contractions. My first experience of the outside world was a violent one. I consider that this experience influenced what would later be my maladaptive choice: Anorexia allowed me to control my own body.

## 3 Impact upon Mothers

Patriarchal silencing of the female voice has not been limited to one generation. Societies teach their constituents the rules of engagement. These rules are passed on from parents to their children, and specific to this discussion, from mothers to their daughters. My voice has been the silenced voice of a daughter, taught by a mother whose voice too was silenced. As women from different generations, our respective rebellions were specific to our contemporary social mandates. Both the relationship of the girl to her social environment and to her mother equally impact her identity development. These interpersonal and socio-political relationships are varied and emotionally complex. They are confusing and conflictual, full of anger, sadness, guilt, blame, frustration, contradiction, and anguish.

The relationship between mothers and daughters is explored by Winnicott (1964) who considers the impact which a baby has upon her mother's sense of independence and freedom. Scholars address the impact which social constructs have had upon the mothers of anorexic daughters:

> Mothers have a right to their anguish, to their conflict, to their doubt and ambivalence and uncertainty about their roles. Why should a woman because she gives birth to a child, cease to be troubled by the profound social and cultural and existential questions? (Chernin, 1985, p. 73)

Mothers silenced and subordinate, pass this socially sanctioned posture of suppression to their daughters. Female anorexia may be a direct response to this patriarchal suppression:

> An eating disorder can be resolved only within the larger cultural context, which allows us to rage because of how terribly we have been mothered

> but including now in this rage, our mothers as daughters with a right to their own despair. Then we shall have liberated an anger that indicts not the mothers but a social system that has never ceased to suppress women. An eating disorder is a profoundly political act. (p. 92)

Hilde Bruch (1973), still considered to be a foremost authority on the emotional aspects of Anorexia Nervosa expresses:

> These women frustrated in the use of their own intellectual abilities and gifts, had become resigned to their fate by the time the anorexic child was born, and had endowed this child with the task of compensating them for their own disappointment. (Holmes, 2016, p. 79)

Contemporary theorists suggest that therapeutic resolve for mothers and daughters involve working together in treatment. The understanding that they share the negative impact of patriarchal suppression and role expectations may encourage a transformation in their relationship and in their own respective identity development:

> The feelings of blame and guilt produce and reinforce feelings of helplessness and powerlessness in mothers and daughters alike, impairing the ability to grow. Although traditional theories suggest that pathology is passed from mother to daughter, a feminist reformulation suggest a different dynamic. Motivated by a desire to remain connected to their mothers, daughters remain unconsciously loyal to their mothers' values and lifestyles. (Rabinor, 1994, p. 277)

Karen (1998) notes that a power struggle between the child and the mother may contribute to the child's developing Anorexia:

> Ambivalent Attachment is a very broad category and can take up residence in the personality in an endless variety of ways but consider the psychological dynamics in some adolescent girls who suffer from Anorexia. Often, the anorectic stance grows directly out of the impossible power relations the child has had with the mother, including feelings of persecution, neglect, and cruelty. In many cases the anorexia develops into an angry refusal not only to take in food but to take in any caring, any emotional nutrition, from another person, even though, deep down, that is what is most wanted. (p. 223)

## 4 Ambivalent Emotions

The paradoxical relationship of loyalty and anger which I experienced toward my mother has confused me. This confusion, brewing for years, remained a silent amber within me. Shame, for many anorexic daughters, has also stoked the fires of their slow burning internal ambivalence:

> A feminist analysis is frequently so liberating for these daughters, who otherwise fail to see themselves as part of a generation struggling for the development their own mothers lacked. They can describe with heartbreaking precision all the suffering their mother endured, broken dreams, failed promises, the hardship and sacrifice of raising children, but it rarely occurs to them that their mother shared this fate with most of the other women of her time. Instead, they tend to explain their mother's life as if they themselves, from earliest infancy, drained and depleted the mother with the intensity of their needs. (Chernin, 1985, p. 64)

## 5 Maternal Feeding

Early maternal feeding styles have also been implicated in the later development of individual and cultural personality styles. Hilde Bruch formulates:

> When a mother learns to offer food in response to signals indicating nutritional needs, the infant will develop the engram[1] of hunger as a sensation distinct from other tensions or needs. However, if the mother's reaction is continuously inappropriate, be it neglectable, over solicitous, inhibiting, or indiscriminately permissive, the outcome for the child will be perplexing confusion in his biological clues and later in his perceptions and conceptualizations. (Sauko, 2008, p. 48)

My mother, gorgeously slender, dropped fourteen-year-old me off at boarding school. Her final words to me were, "This Amish cooking is going to make you really fat." Her motivation was unclear to me. However, I felt that it was cruel, and I responded in my own way to that cruelty. From that day on, not a morsel of that Amish food did I take in.

## 6 Re-Attachment

I have developed a career as an expressive therapist,[2] and for over thirty years have sought to understand and to unravel the puzzling and multidimensional etiology[3] of childhood trauma and the impact which the initial attachment relationship has upon children. It was not until, as an adult, I began to write memoirs based upon my childhood experiences, that I understood how my origin stories impacted my professional life. I worked with diverse groups of children and sought to understand how their social environments and their Psychological Attachment[4] impacted their ability for form healthy relationships. It seems to me that mothers are rerouted away from their instinctive baby rearing knowledge: *Holding the baby, making eye contact, singing to their child.* Many of these instinctive practices have been frowned upon by western doctors and social scientists. They would tell us: Instinct is invisible and cannot be scientifically measured.

My own insecure attachment relationship with my mother motivated me (somewhat unconsciously) to design attachment building programs to help young mothers reclaim their instinctive maternal tools. In the service of illustration, I take a long exhale to describe one of these programs:

Rainbowdance© my attachment enhancing intervention for toddlers, preschool and elementary children, encourages the experience of collective harmony. The beginning ritual circle establishes a sense of containment, safety and empowerment as the children repeat weekly, a sequence of gesture-integrated songs which are easily mastered. Infants express their needs through vocalization and movement. It is this expression that Rainbowdance© assists children of trauma and relocation (adoption and immigration) in recovering. The repetitive content of this intervention assures the establishment of safety, dependability and trust, the necessary precursor to other anticipated goals: promotion of self-esteem, self-regulation, social empathy and, ultimately, healthy relationship building.

The physical relationship of working in circle format promotes attachment through the action of visual and acoustic mirroring, reducing the sense of isolation experienced by children of early trauma and disorganized attachment. The positive experience of moving together, rhythmically lulled by familiar music, contributes to the developing and internalized resource base which children will access in times of conflict or threat. Dynamically moving between affiliation and solitude, the children interact dancing and playing: the retreat into solitude promotes the developing sense of self as each child internalizes the experience of engagement or arousal sequencing. Engagement with a trusting peer group increases the individual and collective competency needed for exploring, risk taking and relationship building. The gross motor component of Rainbowdance© provides children with a symbolic journey into the world of Nature and relationship as they dance the movements of horses, lions and rabbits, and care for the vulnerable baby birds. Following this adventure, children wind down to listen to a soothing story, which provides a smooth transition into the Ending Circle lullaby. Symbolically, children care for babies in the final segment, modeling the care they have received or aspire to receive. This posture promotes the reciprocity of giving and receiving. It encourages the growth of an empowered and self-nurturing child.

When designing this program, I was motivated toward what felt *right* in my body. What felt right was integrating singing with body movement. I chose to give vocal voice to the expressive body voice. I was excited to discover, through research, the neurological and psychological relationships between song and one's perception of safety. This relationship made sense to me: Singing has always been my safe and calming haven. Porges (2011) draws a parallel between the specific tonal frequencies used by composers in writing melodies and that which mothers instinctively use to calm their infants by singing lullabies: "Vocal music triggers neural mechanisms that regulate the entire social engagement system with the resultant changes in facial affect and autonomic state. Basically, we start to look and feel better when we listen to melodies" (pp. 209–210). Lewis et al. (2001) make note of the universality of maternal song: "The limbic brain permits mammals to sing to their children. Vocal communication between a mammal and offspring is universal" (p. 26). In the womb the baby hears the mothers voice and seeks it out after birth. The womb, the original acoustic container of safety, is replicated when the child is sung to. The infant equates the mother's song with safety and will replicate this song for self-soothing in her absence. (Winnicott, 1964). In my program I attempt to replicate this acoustic container of safety with lullaby tunes woven with gentle movements and welcoming gestures. The goal for these groups, where attachments have been severed, inconsistent, or absent, is to help mothers and their children re-attach and to find joy, security, and empowerment in the process.

## Notes

1 a hypothetical permanent change in the brain accounting for the existence of memory; a memory trace. Oxford Dictionary.

2 Expressive arts therapy combines psychology and the creative process to promote emotional growth and healing. www.psychologytoday.com

3 *Psychological etiology* refers to the scientific investigation into the origins of a disorder that cannot be explained biologically. www.encyclopedia.com

4 Attachment refers to *a relationship bond between a child or young person and their primary caregiver*. This bond is formed in the early years and has a long-term impact on a child's sense of self, development, growth and future relationships with others. www.mentallyhealthyschools.org.uk

## References


Albinhac, A. M. H., Jean, F. A. M., & Bouvard, M. P. (2019). Study of parental bonding in childhood in children and adolescents with anorexia nervosa. *L'Encephale, 45*(2), 121–126. https://doi-org.proxy.myunion.edu/10.1016/j.encep.2018.02.004

Bretherton, I. (1992). The origins of attachment theory: John Bowlby and Mary Ainsworth. *Developmental Psychology, 28*(5).

Bruch, H. (1973). *Eating disorders: Obesity, anorexia nervosa, and the person within.* Basic Books, HarperCollins Publishers.

Chernin, K. (1985). *The hungry self: Women, eating and identity*. HarperCollins.

Erikson, E. (1950). *Childhood and society*. W.W. Norton & Company.

Holmes, S. (2016). Between feminism and anorexia: An autoethnography. *International Journal of Cultural Studies, 19*(2), 193–207. https://doi-org.proxy.myunion.edu/10.1177/1367877914561831

Karen, R. (1998). *Becoming attached: First relationships and how they shape our capacity to love.* Oxford University Press.

Lewis, T., Amini, F., & Lannon, R. (2001). *A general theory of love*. Random House, Inc.

Odent, M. (1999). *The scientification of love.* Free Association Books Limited.

Porges, S. (2011). *The polyvagal theory: Neurophysiological foundations of emotions, attachment, communication, self-regulation.* W.W. Norton& Co.

Rabinor, J. (1994). Mothers, daughters, and eating disorders: Honoring the mother daughter relationship. In P. Falloon, M. A. Katzman, & S. C. Wooley (Eds.), *Feminist perspectives on eating disorders*. The Guilford Press.

Saukko, P. (2008). *The anorexic self: A personal and political analysis of a diagnostic discourse.* State University of New York Press.

Scaer, R. C. (2007). *The body bears the burden: Trauma, dissociation, and disease.* Routledge.

Winnicott, D. W. (1964). *The child, the family, and the outside world.* Perseus Publishing.

CHAPTER 3

# Outside

## *Shaping the Scripted Body*

> Just as women used to be unconscious of the powerful effects that cultural stereotypes had on them, they may also be unconscious of powerful forces within them that influence what they do and how they feel.
>
> SHINODA BOLEN (p. 1)

## 1 Introduction

We have ingested the patriarchal voice that devalues women; Our female voices have been silenced both in inward appraisal and in outward expression. We have been told that the knowledge we have amassed through our intuition and through our lived experiences is irrelevant in the patriarchy. So, we will simply do what good girls do, we will follow his rules.

The patriarchy model defines women as *not being good enough;* the hungry young girl devours this definition. She is told that the world sees her as lacking in something. This definition is her first and sustained food. Much of what comes naturally to a woman she will suppress. Anything determined to be *naturally feminine*, she has been taught, is an embarrassment. She adapts her behaviors in accordance with the phallocratic model. Rather than enhancing her innate proclivities (such as creating partnerships, expressing emotion, negotiating, and supporting others), she mimics *his* model. *His* oppositional model placing value upon competing rather than communing. In *his* model there is always a winner and a loser. The drive toward belonging compels women to do as they [the dominant men] do. *Fear* is a by-product of this model, I suggest, because no one wants to lose. And in the patriarchy, women will always lose. Fear is our first emotion (Ekman). Perhaps that is why it is our default, our home base, the familiar.

The culture of patriarchy challenges our innate human relational capacities, those necessary for survival. These capacities, in the gender hierarchy, are undervalued as they are perceived as feminine expressions. Patriarchal hierarchy

 | DOI:10.1163/9789004711051_004

also divides reason from emotion and self from relationships (Gilligan, 2023, p. 16). The feminine, harmonious, communal, emotional is relegated to the box of frivolity. Contrary to this gendered categorization, scientific research, deemed a masculine endeavor, notes that all life forms, from cell to community *need to be in relationship* to thrive. As neuroscientist experts on trauma concur, separations once viewed as signposts of development are now recognized to be manifestations of injury or trauma. "The separation of reason from emotion and of the self from relationship are manifestations of moral injury" (Dossey, p. 82).

The healthy human psyche as well as the social human world demands integration rather than polarization of the two. We women have always known this to be a truth. This truth now spoken through the male voice of science, the measurable, the overt, contradicts the classification of integration as feminine. Relationship building is necessary for the survival all life forms from cells to communities. Sadly, this truth is only acted upon if spoken through a male voice or equivalent entity such as scientific research. This fact reminds me of what often happens to career women in patriarchal cultures; To claim visibility, whether in politics, medicine, or business, they must silence their feminine voices, and alter their personas and expressions to mimic the male version. They still whisper their silenced truths but must morph them to appear acceptably masculine.

We women have been trained to believe that our truths are untruths. Therefore, what lies within, our unconscious material, our knowledge-based power, we hide or disguise. Bringing out unconscious material, that fruit forbidden or made rancid in the patriarchy, with validation, could help us to shift our locus of control; this shift moves the control from the patriarchal external to reclaimed feminine internal. As we act, as we mobilize, we may move forward with agency. This agency, I suggest, brings with it the personal momentum necessary for self-acceptance and for a new perception of fear. We need to experience fear. For in fact, without fear, one cannot develop bravery. We need bravery in our tool kit. It is courage and strength that women must wear as shielding armor against the destructive forces of the patriarchy. "The woman feeling herself seen may learn that she can be seen" (Frye, p. 172). A woman seen, heard, and validated, is a woman who might develop the confidence and agency needed to weather the phallocratic storm and to unleash her true silenced voice.

## 2 Vocally Bipolar

Carole Gilligan (2023) speaks of a split that exists between our two voices: Our *scripted female voice*, our second language which we are taught to express, the one which follows our cognitive learned brain information and secondly, our *native tongue*, our feeling voice, the inner silenced voice which we know is the true voice.[1] She describes how it is that girls learn that if they are honest about their thoughts and feelings, no one will want to be with them. “The price of having relationships was an inner silence” (p. 81). Further she notes:

> Internalization of the gender binary and hierarchy marks the psyches induction into patriarchy. As a rule of thumb, when you hear a gender binary (human capabilities spoken of as either masculine or feminine) and a hierarchy where masculine is elevated over feminine, (reason over emotion, self over relationships), you know you’re in patriarchy, however it may be called. (p. 82)

Jungian psychologist Shinoda Bolen (2014) regarding integration and identity, describes this split as a binocular perception of women psychology:

> There are two powerful forces that shape every woman’s life: the archetypes within us and the outside culture of family society and religion. We need to become conscious about both in order to make informed choices about what we do with our one precious life. (Shinoda Bolen, 2014, p. XVIII)

We women are split into many pieces: our voices within and the multitude of competitive voices without. We girls, looking for guidance for our identity development, dissociate or hallucinate, to survive being lost in the cacophony of conflicting messages. Social binarism discounts all the metaphorical gray area existent between the extremes of black and white. The reduction of cause and effect to good or bad social scenarios sustain the binarism of dominance and subordination.

Binarism is the default that we have historically internalized. Beyond the restrictive polarity of black and white lies the unexplored domain of integration. Moving into the unexplored takes the courage we need as individuals and as a society to change our perception of gender with its restrictions and its manifestations. The problem is that we ALL, men and women must dive within to affect any change. We ALL have both black and white within. The self-accepting individual still needs to confront a social and political environment which is hostile or condescending. Societal change of this perception required an “excavation of the patriarchal model of dominance and subordination” (S. Bolen).

Social belonging is a primary goal for coming-of-age adolescents; prerequisite to achieving this goal is the formation of a secure personal identity. Adolescents look to trusted adults to help them interpret the necessary credentials for social acceptance. *I want to belong, so I follow the rules*. However, there are more than one set of rules. As a teen girl, I experienced ambivalent messages; I internalized these mixed messages from my social, familial, and political environments:

> Look to your mother for guidance. Find a better role model. Pretend that he is your father not the one in Pennsylvania. Don't forsake your true paternity. Get good grades at all costs. Being happy is more important than academic success. Smile and pretend. Get angry and fight.

With no clear direction, I kept quiet. As a child I had been fed too many dissonant messages. This conflict from the social environment contributed to my identity ambivalence. In this confusion, one message was clear: A woman's way of knowing and her life experiences have little value in my world. Today social and political conflicts, like cancers, are metastasizing. Our world is providing its youth with continued and growing identity confusion.

## 3 Body Politics: Female and Nature

I draw attention to the distinction between the perception of *image* and *body* for its impact upon identity development and cultural belonging. The former is two-dimensional, the later, three-dimensional. One is superficial, the other alive. The psychological conflict between the interpretation and identity experience of the two amplifies the already existent ambivalence and confusion for the coming-of-age girl. She is told that *image,* not *body* (female), is to be valued. The media describes that socially acceptable image. This conflict, one facet in the diverse and discordant tapestry of mixed social messages represents a harbinger for coming-of-age confusion:

> Being in a body means feeling hunger and desire, satiation and frustration, pleasure, and pain. An image is created when someone is looking. An image is flat, it has no feeling, is silent. An image can have no appetite, no hunger, no desire, and no power of its own. An image creates a 'no-body body', nobody's body because we exist not in images that reflect others' desires but in desiring bodies… Knowledge is power. The knowledge that girls and women who hold in their bodies is a source of power that the image of the desirable woman obscures. (Tolman & Debolt, p. 301)

Much of what defines *female* cannot be seen: from her reproductive organs to her unconscious ruminations. Because it is beyond his control, the male, the king fears what he cannot see. I posit that *natural* and *not real* are similar by male definition, both of which define the woman. (He values only what he creates). In a world where validation is not forthcoming, the woman has developed an identity that reflects the inferiority awarded to her by her dominators. Forced to mimic the dominant white male model, she (and other marginalized groups) has made covert her own ideals and beliefs. By virtue of the act of mimicry, this superficial expression of *his* knowledge, untrue to *her* own, renders it *inferior*. And, she has learned that her truth, her inner voice, is also inferior. So, in the patriarchy, what she expresses and what she silences are both equally unworthy. "Patriarchy depends for its continuation on violence and on silence" (Gilligan, 2023, p. 18).

The expression of contemporary Body Politics has been reshaped by the American feminist perspective:

> Feminism inverted and converted the old metaphor of the Body Politic found in Plato, Aristotle, etc. to a new metaphor: the politics of the body. In the old metaphor of the Body Politic, the state or society was imagined as a human body, with different organs and parts symbolizing different functions, needs, social constituents and forces, the head or soul for the sovereign, the blood for the will of the people, or the nerves for the system of rewards and punishments. Now feminism imagined the human body as *itself* a politically inscribed entity, its physiology and morphology shaped by histories and practices of containment and control, from foot binding and corseting to rape and battering to compulsory, heterosexuality, forced sterilization, unwanted pregnancy, and explicit commodification. (Bordo, 1993, p. 21)

Consider the role that the material and metaphorical female body plays in contemporary body politics. The female and her body have always, in the Western patriarchal designed theatre, been associated with the less valued entity. She is of the earth, she is feeling, she is abstract, she is covert, she is not worthy of participating in his discourse. She has been relegated to the roles that he designed for her, all in the service of maintaining his dominance. These roles suppress her strengths as they force her to behave in a manner that she *knew* is false:

> Female bodies have historically been significantly more vulnerable than male bodies to extremes in both forms of cultural manipulation of the body. Perhaps this has something to do with the fact that women, besides *having* bodies, are also *associated* with the body, which has always been considered woman's "sphere" in family life, in mythology, in scientific, philosophical, and religious ideology. (Bordo, 1993, p. 143)

A culture that associates women with their bodies, prompts coming-of-age females to take control and shape those bodies as vehicles for surrendering and gaining entre into that society. The distinction can be drawn between *willing* to surrender to patriarchal scripting and the *will* needed to exert control over the body: "I've learned to be a stronger person with a more powerful will… pure concentration, energy and spirit" (Bordo, p. 98). By *willing*, Bordo refers to the way in which girls exercise the power that has been made available to them-exhibiting the power of weakness and internalization of mechanisms of their own oppression. C. Gilligan (1982) and R. Solnit (2017) advocated for the inclusion of the literal and metaphorical feminine voice in all discourses:

> Silence is what allows people to suffer without recourse, what allows hypocrisies and lies to grow and flourish, crimes to go unpunished. If our voices are essential aspects of our humanity, to be rendered voiceless is to be dehumanized or excluded from one's humanity. And the history of silence is central to women's history. (Solnit, p. 18)

By restricting their voices, many women are wittingly or unwittingly perpetuating a male-voiced civilization and an order of living that is founded on disconnection from women (Gilligan, 1980, p. XI).

Christine Caldwell, a dance movement therapist and educator, considers body equity and the relationship of the individual female body to the social body:

> Body equity need not only involve unraveling the *less-than* status of the body as it is compared with the mind, and the falsehood of seeing them as separate… We can examine our clinical assumptions about the quiet, or slumped, or aggressive, or tense body as well through the lens of social theory this body might be taking the only shape that society will allow it. (p. 283)

## 4 Why Females Experience Highest Rates of Anorexia Nervosa

Varied theories explicate how gender differences, both biological and sociological, might be implicated in the disproportionate rate of anorexia in females. The theories link patriarchal scripting of women as subservient with the development of this disorder. Scaer (2007) suggests that women assume familiar patriarchal roles of helplessness and experience guilt and self-blame. I suggest that this expression has become the norm for patriarchal women, and that Anorexia is one of many reactions to the role that positions them toward self-deprecation. On another note, because the body of the female is culturally devalued, the young girl may take possession of what society renders disposable, her female body. She eats and reshapes the discarded crumbs.

Another theory suggested that female fasting might be equated with religious purity. Religion, being abstract, is a product of the human imagination, one which creates myth stories. Faith places value upon what is unseen; The unseen, the imagined, resides in the realm of female sensibility. She might be more inclined than is he, to engage in religious rituals, such as starvation. This ritual is historic in Western culture, dating back to the female medieval saints. Brumberg (1988) suggest that an element of this association continues: "In different times women fasting has had different meanings. Still in the 19th century fasting women were understood by themselves and their audiences in terms of religious miracles, purity, and chastity" (Saukko, 2008, p. 17).

During the period of my own anorexia, I did experience a purity and an exaggerate sense of spirituality. During that time, I believe that my spiritual purity was resultant rather than precursory to my starvation. I would see visions that made me feel otherworldly and unusual. I was no longer ordinary. I was no longer following the patriarchal and otherwise external rules. I had gained control in a world that seemed out of my control, and I felt as if I was floating above that world. I was terrified to fall from this grace. The falling, I believed would occur if I started to eat again.

## 5 Patriarchal: Social Expectations and Media Influence

Scholars continue to explore how cultural artifacts, such as music, architecture, visual imagery, film, and fashion, have fortified feminine passivity and subordination in the patriarchal script. The female image generated by the media *machine* through the vehicle of public consciousness, is fed into one's social consciousness and one's developing identity. The little girl looks to the world around her for direction. She assumes that the messages she received will fortify her developing identity and assist her in establishing her place in a welcoming world. She wants to belong. In the patriarchy, those messages have been designed primarily by men. These designs shape and script women into submissive roles which support continued male dominance. These are the designs that children of the 1960s were exposed to. In the service of developing autonomy and self-control, this mimicking was later followed by rebellious rejection. The cultural messages internalized by coming-of-age girls, reflected time-specific political, scientific, and social agenda. Hilda Bruch (1978) attacks post-war mass-culture middle-class domesticated femininity of the 50s and 60s. "Bruch demonstrates that our current understanding of Anorexia as having to do with a lack of autonomous self-will does not indicate a psychological universal but is deeply lodged in a specific historical place and time and its political agenda" (Saukko, p. 10). Orbach (1993) additionally notes the significance of early parenting and of perceived belonging:

> The rise in the incidence of Anorexia Nervosa provides us with an unusually visible example of the way in which psychic structure and symptom formation are determined by three factors: the social climate of a period; particular models of parenting; and the attempt of each generation to find its place in the world. (p. 12)

## 6 Beauty Ideal

The media's presentation of the ideal female form had changed over time reflecting respective social and political climates. Girls coming of age in the mid 1960s were overwhelmed with transitional and changing images of ideal feminine beauty and the medias depiction of that ideal. Contradictions have existed and still exist in the western cultural meaning of slenderness. The "many layers of cultural significance are crystalized in this disorder" (Bordo, 1993, p. 67). Adolescents look to the media for the acceptable beauty ideal. During my teen years the media displayed consistently diverse, rapidly changing, and conflictual ideals.

The era following World War Two, the "fuller figure", as Jane Russell called it, came into fashion once more, a period of "mammary madness (or resurgent Victorianism as Lois Banner called it), which glamorized the voluptuous large-breasted woman. This remained the prevailing fashion tyranny until the late 1960s and early 1970s" (Bordo, p. 159) followed by the wave of British fashion ideals. Twiggy, with her thin boy-like body, became the new physical model for girls to emulate: the frail, almost emaciated skinny female. A similarity between the 1920s and the 1960s ideals, both eras in which women's movements were erupting, could be noted: "In the 1920s, young women began to flatten their breasts, sucking their stomachs, bobbing their hair, and showing long colt-like legs. They believed they were pursuing a new freedom and daring that demanded a carefree, boyish style" (Ibid., p. 163).

The media's mixed messages may also contribute to girls' anxieties about growing up:

> Anorexics do not want to grow up to mature womanhood. Feminists see anorexia as a contradiction; the women are at the same time conforming to the ideal of feminine beauty and rebelling against it. This anxiety over the female body can be understood as rebellion against limiting gender roles. But it can also aim at suppressing the archetypal negative. (Sauko, 2008)

"Of course, from birth to puberty the little girl grew up, but never felt growth; Day after day her body was present like an exact finished thing; Now she is developing. The very word horrifies her" (de Beauvoir, p. 320).

It is the change in her body that marks this transition. She sees it when she looks in the mirrors, both physical and social. It is this change that she attempts to slow down or halt. She wants to remain the child who was taken care of and was not aware of restrictive social mandates and rules. Awareness of these restrictions, I suggest, might cause her to seek freedom from their mandates. Returning to the body of her childhood might be a solution. She attempts at slowing down her biological development, of the physical body she inhabits. This body which classifies her as *female,* she attempts to control. She is determined to resist progressing into the social category of *woman.* She may starve herself to remain physically small. She wants to feel a sense of control over her embodied destiny and what it implies regarding her social destiny. Her body is tangible; society is an abstract. She is repulsed by the roles that she sees her mother and other women playing. She does not want to join the club designed wherein its members sustain the dominant cultural framework:

> I wanted to grow up, but never did I seriously dream of leading the life I saw adults lead… And the desire to grow up without ever assuming an adult state, without ever feeling solidarity with parents, mistresses of the house, housewives, or heads of family, was forming in me. (de Beauvoir, p. 336)

I can't remember if my aversion to the voluptuous female images presented in Playboy like girly magazines was fueled by my fear of growing up (and all the associated responsibilities) or a personal dislike for that aesthetic. I only know that, at all costs, I did not want to be full figured. The media's new waiflike boyish models supported my waning physical body. Among other influences and directives, I sensed that looking small and needy would categorize me as one to be cared for rather than as a caretaker. Claiming control in a situation where all else had been taken from me, I stopped eating. Chiseled down to bare bone, I left my boarding school and found that, when I returned home to my local school I was treated like a celebrity. Everyone wanted to take care of me or to have me model for their photographs or fashion shows. I was no longer ordinary but rather viewed as extraordinary. The origin of my starvation was not based upon the new beauty ideal; However, the media valued and supported my new skinny body. It was difficult for me to give that up. I was finally adored; my body finally had a voice that was deemed worthy of listening to.

## 7 Music

Music provided subliminal and overt messages supportive of patriarchal scripting for women and girls during my 1960s childhood.[2] The voice of the individual woman was muffled by the wave of the scripted happy housewife in post-World War Two America. Partly responsible for this muffling, I argue, were contemporary song lyrics, specifically those of Burt Bacharach and Hal David. My understanding, as I recall the mothers of the 1960's, is that Bacharach type music provided an acoustic ball and chain. It confined women within the fenced boundaries of their *Happy Housewife* script. This script, socially ascribed "a set of instructions for what women and men must do in order to be happy, whereby happiness is what follows being natural or good" (Ahmed, 2010, p. 59). Their music was a constant in my childhood home. We, the daughters, did not yet know we were role playing in the patriarch theatre. Literal was our interpretation of the lyrics. The songs became our Bibles, our road maps to becoming. I heard these at the age of five, could sing them without prompt by age eight, and remember them verbatim today:

> Hey! Little girl
> Comb your hair, fix your makeup
> Soon he will open the door
> Don't think because there's a ring on your finger
> You needn't try anymore.
> For wives should always be lovers too
> Run to his arms the moment he comes home to you
> I'm warning you (Bacharach, David, 1963).

The historic and intergenerational script has been passed, with the help of such music, from mother to daughter. More boisterous music (such as Jazz or the newly coming to us, Rock) was perceived as a threat to the patriarchal status quo. Such music might fuel the fires of female rebellion.

Second wave feminism began in 1963, the year that Bacharach's song was made popular. This wave focused on achieving equality and opportunities for women without the constraints of gender expectations. The British cultural wave swept America in the 1960s, transforming the 1950s American fashion and beauty ideals, as well as the musical standard. The new lyrics sang of freedom and joy, juxtaposing a new potential upon the established 1950s lounge music. The Beatles had just arrived on the music scene.

Bacharach's listening audience was primarily female. The singers were primarily male. However, Dionne Warwick, a Black woman, popularized Bacharach's music, even singing one rendition of Wives *and Lovers* (whose lyrics are cited above). It is interesting to consider that as the songbird, the harbinger of this message, she, a Black woman, spoke to white privileged housewives encouraging them to remain subordinate. Karen Carpenter, a white female vocalist who also popularized much of Bacharach music, became anorexic and finally, committed suicide. She sang the scripted patriarchal song and suffocated on her silenced voice:

> Karen collapsed in Las Vegas in 1975 while singing *Top of the World*, an event which began to open to public consciousness the condition of Anorexia Nervosa. An upbeat country-tinged love song *Top of the World* had been a No.1 single in the United States in 1973 and was a highlight of the Carpenters' live show. The opening line is *Such a Feeling Coming over Me* (Carpenters 1972)—if not dissociated, is this what you sing before your body collapses on stage? (McKay, 2018, p. 6)

Regarding this persona and its repressed underbelly, Saukko (2008) reflects:

> Being middle class and being good or perfect, characteristics associated with the Carpenters, were often conflated with the diagnostic criteria of Anorexia… she was associated with freshness and youth and stood in opposition to the masculine, rough, Hard Rock, associated with political protest in the drug culture of the era.
>
> Carpenter's death from Anorexia was harnessed to reveal the psychologically and politically repressive underside of 1970s political neo-conservatism. (pp. 65, 67)

The music and those that voiced it were supportive of and impacted by the patriarchal script.

## 8 Stories and TV

French feminist, Simone de Beauvoir (2011) notes the existent problem of media's negative impact upon female identity during her lifetime (original manuscript dated 1949). She explores the relationship of the female body to identity and to the myth of the eternal feminine. She questions and offers insight into the question, "why women do not contest male sovereignty" and "where the submission in women comes from" (p. 7). She traces the social and emotional development of the girl from infancy to adulthood. She notes the impact that childhood stories and images have upon identity (p. 302), especially regarding the subliminal identity reinforcement of feminine subordination and passivity.

Inconsistencies between the depiction of middle-class homes are apparent in 1960s TV and film. This inconsistency contributed to the tapestry of social mixed messages:

> The middle-class family and its central character, the mother, were a politically loaded subject in the Cold War period. On one hand, the newly affluent ranch house and refrigerator family with his homemaker mother was used as proof of the superiority of the American system of morals, politics, and economics. On the other hand, the suburban home became a source of cultural agony. Amidst early TV dramas that embraced family values such as *Father Knows Best* there were movies that depicted the middle-class home as a loveless place reigned over by passive aggressive mothers devouring their children such as the James Dean films. (Saukko, p. 49)

*Father Knows Best* was the model for family dynamics offered by my parents. I did not see James Dean films until I was an adult. Secrets prevailed, especially regarding models that would challenge our designated scripts. Such secrets underline what the media presents and what the curious adolescent is still hungry to explore.

## 9 Glamorization and Mimicry: Social Media

The media offers many vehicles through which imitation and glamorization of Anorexia continue to occur. I witnessed and was horrified by such a 1980's glamorization of Anorexia. A TV movie had been made in which the protagonist was a beautiful female teen anorexic. I remembered thinking, because of my own anorectic experience, that this was going to bring with it tremendous harm, specifically in the form of imitation. The experience was glamorized, and teens, it was reported, did imitate the heroine (because the protagonist, regardless of her story, was in the media, and therefore, worthy of imitation):

"Sunday night TV movies such as *For the Love of Nancy* and *Dying to be Perfect*, and underground films such as *Superstar: the Karen Carpenter Story* as well as talk shows, psychiatric journals, textbooks, treatment regimens and feminist research on the condition" (Saukko, p. 54) popularize the anorexic as a heroine.

Celebrities with eating disorders further popularize and intensify this potential for mimicry. The celebrity stories of Karen Carpenter (previously discussed) and Princess Diana during my adolescence I offer as examples:

> The media coverage of the two celebrities draws attention to the fact that the popular discourses on thinness and popular discourses on eating disorders are very similar, fomenting women's anxieties about not being strong and independent enough or not being adaptive and caring enough. The politically invested news stories on Carpenter and Princess Diana underline the influence of broad social structures and agendas-rather than just media enthusiasm with thinness-on popular discourses and attendant behavioral norms on how women should relate to their selves, their bodies, and the world. (Saukko, 2008, p. 58)

The media, especially the contemporary social media, provides examples for beauty and success that immature girls mimic. The media has been selective in choosing its heroines. I suggest that primarily the rich and famous have been historically (since the development of social media) brought to our attention. Anorexia is presented as one of the vehicles for becoming as *fabulous an image as* media *role* models.

The patriarchal model continues to increase its stronghold on Western media. Children have increased access to digital and technical communication tools and, consequently, to patriarchal media. *We want to be what we see. We want to belong.*

Patriarchal-designed identity, as I hope this book reveals, is destructive. As scholars, parents, and educators, we are positioned to influence what children are exposed to. Consequently, we are positioned to assist this next generation of coming-of-age girls (and boys) towards empowered and healthy identities, and towards social justice. Additionally, we must consider the impact of digital relationship building upon contemporary identity development as technology increases rather than decreases as the default method for communication. This is an important consideration now as children experience increased isolation and dependance upon technology following the Covid-19 pandemic. Current research investigates the recent rise in eating disorders among children: "The COVID-19 pandemic has had considerable mental health consequences for children and adolescents, including the exacerbation of previously diagnosed eating disorders" (Agostino et al., 2020, p. 1). I suggest an exploration into the relationship between isolation and the rise in eating disorders.

## 10 Isolation: Fuel or Extinguish the Anorexic Fire

Medical model remedies for Anorexia include isolation and rest. The prototype for this remedy appeared to date back to Freud who described this cure for women *suffering* from hysteria:

> Freud was blind to the contribution that isolation, boredom, and intellectual frustration made to the etiology of hysteria. Nearly all of his subjects he acknowledged to be unusually intelligent, creative, energetic, independent and often, highly educated. So too for the anorectic it is indeed essential to recognize in this illness the dimension of protest against limitations of the ideal female domesticity (the 'Feminine Mystique' as Betty Friedan called it) that reigned in America throughout the 1950s and 1960s, the era when most of their mothers were starting homes and families. (Bordo, 1993, p. 159)

This forced isolation, supportive of the Western medical model, perpetuates the notion that women must be controlled to be healthy. "Psychiatry ends up as an accomplice to the same cruel sociocultural processes that inform anorexia. It fights its patients with their own method, control, deepening it" (Saukko, 2008, p. 20). As I had experienced it, control had been exerted upon me, truncating my ability to self-control. This catalyzed a battle of wills: *who would gain control over my body?* I experienced this battle of wills as a struggle to outsmart the medical providers. Medical treatment of anorexia, donning a mask of helping, conceals it true violence:

> Clinical, popular, and even feminist discourses on anorexia seem to help anorexics by enabling them to regain weight and health without addressing the underlying psychological and familial issues, harmful discourses, and gendered inequalities. The trouble with this 'helping' is that it masks the sheer violence and disrespect embedded in the way in which anorexics are treated in psychiatric environments. (Saukko, p. 33)

When I was anorexic, I equated isolation with self-control. In an isolated environment I was in control, disengaged from family and mealtime. There,

I felt I was able to have the fortitude necessary to starve myself and stay on course. I became anorexic again when in another isolated environment (college). Therefore, I suggest that isolation might amplify the expression of Anorexia. In an isolated environment the only voice one hears is her own. The mixed and chaotic messages expressed from outside are silenced. This is especially relevant today as research shows that female teenage Anorexia has increased during the isolation forced upon us by the Covid pandemic.

## 11 Contemporary Social Media

Bringing us up to date, I venture into the world of contemporary social media. Digital relationships perpetuate social and relational isolation: one sees and takes in a message but there is no requirement to respond, no call and response of live engagement. In her book *Perfect: Feeling judged on social media,* Gill (2023) advises: "Compared with previous generations, today's young women live in a world where visual images of women's bodies are ubiquitous in media, public space and especially online" (p. 3). She further forewarns of the danger inherent to this exposure in its "way of seeing among young women-the extraordinary level of detail apprehended in just a momentary glance noting that this mode of seeing subsumes the hostile, evaluative judging gaze that many women themselves feared" (p. 174). There is no potential to question or to respond to what is shown. Disempowerment.

Current research into the impact of social media, specifically Instagram and Tik Tok reveals its relationship to eating disorders and to other adolescent mental health identity issues. Researchers found that:

> Significant relationships emerged between the frequency of Instagram use and body dis-satisfaction, drive for thinness and low self-esteem in adolescents and young adults (14–24 years), and between the frequency of Instagram use and drive for thinness in the older age group (25–35 years). Thus, continuing modifications in the use of SM by children and adolescents may potentially lead to the development of disordered eating cognition and eating disorders in new generations. (Pruccoli, 2022, p. 6)

Women are taught repeatedly to see themselves through the lens of imperfection. With access to and obsession with continued reference to social media, there no peace from this message. To keep up with what is happening requires never tuning out. Girls are bombarded with unnatural presentations of beauty, which they are told simultaneously or subliminally, they will never live up to. The superficial rather than the deep is valued. What you see becomes what you are. Recently a friend, a plastic surgeon told me that young girls choose to alter their faces and bodies to mimic the unnatural depicted on social media even though in "real life" they look like monsters. Priority is given to their digital rather than face to face image. Isolation is promoted. Interactive engagement is truncated. Life forms, I remind you, according to science, die in isolation.

I watch twelve- and thirteen-year-old girls that I know, mimic the sexualized postures, extreme makeup, and scantily clad media models. They attempt to replicate what they see. They do not, I believe, understand the sexual nature of these *role models*. They are not trying to be sexy to get boys to notice them, they are simply trying to look like what they see. They are desperate to belong, to not be excluded. To be enough.

> A pressing need exists to understand the complex nature and conflicting characteristics of SM usage, and to fully explore how a relationship with SM, whether actively sought or accepted through passive exposure, can influence a sensitive population group such as our young and adolescent patients with regard to body image concerns and eating disturbances. (Pruccoli, p. 3)

Girls need to have therapeutic, educational, and creative supports to help them interpret what the media displays. Healthy navigation, for the coming-of-age girl, requires from the social environment those ingredients that were necessary for early attachment: consistency, responsiveness, sustainment, and support. I believed that throughout life we continually require this foundation for security at our crossroads. It is risky to leap forward into the unknown; security within and without give us the courage to leap. Every transition presented a doorway. We experienced the doorway as blocked or open. We revisit our need for secure attachment at every transition or turning point. The society that offered this support via rituals and rites of passage presented the doorway as open. Sadly, patriarchal cultures do not open doors for women and girls. However, within the Patriarchy there are women such as me, that are working to educate and guide our young progeny. I found this entry on Facebook this past winter:

> *Imagine something embarrassing happened to you at school when you were in the 7th grade. Everyone laughed and it was awful, and you were mortified. Then a few weeks passed and everybody found new things to laugh about and they moved on. You didn't forget how embarrassed you were, but you could move on too.*

*Now imagine you did something embarrassing in 7th grade. And everyone laughed and it was awful. But someone also caught it on Snapchat. And turned it into a meme. And a Tik Tok. And took a screenshot of it. And spread it further. And you couldn't get away from it. And no one forgot. And you couldn't either. And people were still sharing it months later.*

*Just sit there and imagine it for a minute.*

*Kids aren't ready for social media. It starts with us parents. Please share.* ♥

(Kathy Ahern Lafferty, 2023)

## Notes

1 My terms for these voices.

2 In the 1970s, the popular music industry developed a cult of anorexia, according to George McKay's (2018) "Skinny Blues: Karen Carpenter, Anorexia Nervosa and Popular Music".

## References

Agostino, H., Burstein, B., Moubayed, D., Taddeo, D., Grady, R., Vyver, E., Dimitropoulos, G., Dominic, A., & Coelho, J. S. (2021). Trends in the incidence of new-onset anorexia nervosa and atypical anorexia nervosa among youth during the COVID-19 pandemic in Canada. *JAMA Network Open*, *4*(12), e2137395. https://doi-org.proxy.myunion.edu/10.1001/jamanetworkopen.2021.37395

Ahmed, S. (2010). Feminist killjoys. In *The promise of happiness*. Duke University Press.

Bacharach, B., & David, H. (1963). *Wives and Lovers lyrics* © Sony/ATV Music Publishing LL. (1967). *I Say a Little Prayer lyrics* © Sony/ATV Music Publishing LL.

Bordo, S. (1993). *Unbearable weight: Feminism, western culture and the body*. University of California Press.

Bruch, H. (1973). *Eating disorders: Obesity, anorexia nervosa, and the person within*. Basic Books, HarperCollins Publishers.

De Beauvoir, S. (2011). *The second sex* (1st ed.). Vintage Books.

Frye, M. (1983). To be and be seen: The politics of reality. In *The politics of reality*. The Crossing Press.

Gill, R. (2023). *Perfect: Feeling judged on social media*. Polity Press.

Gilligan, C. (2023). *In a human voice*. Harvard University Press.

Lafferty, K. (2023). Facebook.

McKay, G. (2018). Skinny blues: Karen Carpenter, anorexia nervosa and popular music. *Popular Music*, *37*(1), 1–21. https://doi-org.proxy.myunion.edu/10.1017/S026114301700054X

Orbach, S. (1986). *Hunger strike: The anorectic's struggle as a metaphor for our age.* Faber & Faber.

Pruccoli, J., Marta De Rosa, M., Chiasso, L., Perrone, A., & Parmeggiani, A. (2022).The use of TikTok among children and adolescents: Experience in a third-level public Italian center during the SARS-CoV-2 pandemic. *Italian Journal of Pediatrics, 48*(138).

Saukko, P. (2008). *The anorexic self: A personal and political analysis of a diagnostic discourse.* State University of New York Press.

Scaer, R. C. (2007). *The body bears the burden: Trauma, dissociation, and disease.* Routledge.

Shinoda Bolen, J. (2014). *Goddesses in everywoman: Powerful archetypes in women's lives.* Harper.

Solnit, R. (2017). *The mother of all questions.* Haymarket Books.

Tolman, D., & Debold, E. (1994). Conflicts of body and image: Female adolescence, desire, and the nobody body. In P. Falloon, M. A. Katzman, & S. C. Wooley (Eds.), *Feminist perspectives on eating disorders.* The Guilford Press.

CHAPTER 4

# Choosing Anorexia

*The Vocal Body*

> For us to reject the insistence that a woman's appearance is her speech… is itself a political move forward.
>
> WOLF (p. 275)

## 1 Introduction

The definition, interpretation and treatment of Anorexia Nervosa has been transformed, reshaped, defined, and treated, over time. *Analogous* to consider: The *society* has taken control, reshaped and transformed the definition; the *anorexic* has taken control, reshaped and transformed her body in the process.

In 1945 Ludwig Binswanger noted in the case of Ellen West. "From a psychiatric point of view, we are dealing here with something new, with a new symptom barely known a century ago, now of epidemic proportions" (Bordo, p. 140). In 1973 Hilda Bruch (a pioneer in the understanding and treating of eating disorders) "could still say that Anorexia was rare indeed" (ibid.). Yet in 1984, "1 in every 200 to 250 women between the ages of 13 and 22 suffer from Anorexia. Ninety percent of all anorexics are women" (ibid.). Today female Anorexia, especially following COVID, is on the rise (Agostino et al., 2020, p. 1). As the disorder continues to seek definition, I offer historical interpretations and let this book and my personal experience navigate the reader toward their own understanding of the condition.

For the past one hundred years in western phallocratic societies, many white middle-class girls have chosen Anorexia as a vehicle for mobilization away from the passive postures ascribed to them. Studies have shown that in such societies, female anorexics struggle against feeling enslaved, exploited, and not being permitted to lead lives of their choosing. This book references the historical evolution of Anorexia Nervosa, specifically focusing upon female identity development during the 1960s and 1970s.

 | DOI:10.1163/9789004711051_005

Scholars note consistencies between the social and political backgrounds of the 1920s and the 1960s and their respective expressions of Anorexia. Early feminist authors during the time of Second Wave feminism observe "a considerable rise in eating disorders, [which] linked the problem to the consequences of the Women's Movements the resulting contradictions and pressures surrounding the female role" (Holmes, 2016, p. 7).

As one of those girls that chose Anorexia in the 1960s, rebelling against patriarchal scripting, I suggest that consistencies might be found in the early childhood environments of the later to be anorexic daughters. Music, television, movies, stories, images, home furnishings and fashion wrapped subliminal messaging around women who were mothers, smothering them into submission. I posit that in their desire to please, the daughters drank the Kool-Aid, modeling themselves after their mothers. Daughters of these mothers were passed the scripted torch of devotion. As Simone de Beauvoir (2011) suggests:

> The girl will be wife, mother, grandmother; She will take care of her house exactly as her mother does, she will take care of her children as she was taken care of: she is twelve years old and her story is already written in the heavens; She will discover day after day without shaping it she is curious but frightened when she thinks about this life whose every step is planned in advance and toward which every day irrevocably moves her. (p. 312)

## 2 Treatment

Anorexia Nervosa has been defined in clinical, feminist, and popular discourses. Through the feminist lens, Anorexia is understood to be a reaction to the social oppression of women in Western culture. The medical model defines the etiology as biological or neurological. Medical model interventions and treatments overlook the impact of social oppression, the anorexic's early attachment scenario and her consequent emotional makeup. Understanding the true multi-faceted etiology of the disorder must incorporate all concepts of the literal and metaphorical "inside and outside." These included the following influences: (1) the original maternal relationship, inclusive of the impact of the patriarchy upon mothers, (2) the relationship between the anorexic and her socio-political environment, and (3) the impact of the patriarchy upon discourses and treatment of Anorexia Nervosa.

I have gravitated toward those scholars who advocate for listening to, rather than speaking for, the female anorexic. Historically, her opinions on the definitions and treatments of her disorder have been disregarded. This disregard,

I believe, represents the general disregard for the female voice in the Western patriarchal society. Susie Orbach (Bordo, 1993) defines AN as part of a female continuum: "Anorexia represents one extreme on a continuum of which all women today find themselves, insofar as they are vulnerable, to one degree or another, to the requirements of the cultural construction of femininity" (p. 47). Further Orbach suggests: "Anorexia appears less as the extreme expression of a character structure [of culture] than as a remarkably overdetermined symptom of some of the multifaceted and heterogeneous distresses of our age" (Ibid., p. 141).

The contemporary medical and psychiatric perspective describe Anorexia Nervosa as biologically or genetically based. The Anorexic is perceived in this (patriarchal) model, to be damaged, to need external control, to be unworthy of participating in her own treatment. Current treatments[1] continue to advocate for maintenance of medically based behavioral control over patients, rather than providing them with tools for understanding the emotional and social etiology of the disorder.

Feminist interpretations, on the other hand, view eating disorders as reactions to the social oppression of women in western culture.[2] By definition, oppression presumes a dynamic of perpetrator and victim, a battle for command or control. My lived experience as a teen anorexic gives me the standpoint to make the following statement: Treatments based upon the western medical perspective have the potential to amplify rather than diminish the symptoms associated with Anorexia Nervosa. "Psychiatry ends up as an accomplice to the same cruel sociocultural processes that inform anorexia. It fights its patients with their own method, control, deepening it" (Saukko, 2008, p. 20). I had experienced such a battle.

Understanding the emotional and social etiology of anorexia might assist patients and medical providers in choosing constructive rather than destructive psychological and physical control mechanisms and treatments.

Historically, female psychiatric disorders such as depression, headaches, nervousness, self-doubt, and hysteria were treated by male doctors with the *rest cure* (Bordo, 1988). Any display of female emotion was treated with this *cure*. Freud laid the foundation for such psychiatric treatment and was "blind to the contribution that isolation, boredom, and intellectual frustration made in the etiology of hysteria" (Bordo, p. 104). Scholars, clinicians, and historians draw parallels between the etiology and historical treatment of both hysteria and anorexia.

The patriarchal notion that females are damaged or broken and must be fixed and controlled through a science-based regimen has been sustained throughout history. This regime disempowers the anorexic and disregards her motivation toward positive identity development: "So long as eating disorders remain situated within a medical model, those who are entrusted with the conceptualization of anorexia and bulimia will be the medical professionals who have little experience in or inclination towards cultural interpretations and criticism" (p. 69).

Barrows (2021) distrusted the behavioral treatment which the medical model prescribed for his anorexic wife. Rather than attempting to force her into this treatment, he entered their relationship as an emotional peer. His *cure* was to love rather than to save her. He chose to engage in a relationship rather than in isolating her. Control over her actions and her body were hers, not his, he believed. Ultimately, she slowly, found her own way back to health. Love, respect, and validation rather than usurped control was her medicine. Loss of control or power, I believe, is an underlying issue for anorexics. Saukko (2008), also a former anorexic, emphasizes the value found in listening to the stories of those who the medical model continues to blindly and unsuccessfully treat:

> It is my aim to fight back against the tendency to silence anorexic women's criticism of their treatment and the way in which they are described in public media, and to underline the need to listen to anorexic women's views of the discourses and practices that are allegedly helping them. (p. 34)

This book offers, via my memoir, my views, my stories.

## 3 Rites of Passage into Womanhood

Cultural rituals have lost their value and consequent placement in Western patriarchal traditions. Those that honor and assist girls for transitioning into womanhood are essentially nonexistent. Recognizing this significant gap, I have created arts-based workshops that include rites of passage rituals for woman and girls. In retrospect, I understand that these cultural rituals were absent during my own coming of age.

Chernin (1985) differentiates rites of passage in traditional and indigenous cultures from those of modern western cultures. She notes that rites of initiation are of primary importance in traditional societies, while they are practically non-existent in the modern western world. The purpose of traditional rites of passage are twofold: "the transformation of identity and the entry into culture" (p. 166). Rituals involving food and the body are foundational to most traditional transition rites, as are separation of the girl from the mother. The traditional restricting of food intake as part of these rites of passage have religious or spiritual foundations. Although modern western girls who restrict their food intake may mimic some of these traditional rituals of passage, they are doing so without the spiritual or religious associations of the rituals. While food denial may have been a personally empowering act, without its cultural and religious meanings, the denial would not assist them in entering their culture (the second benefit of traditional food denial); Fruitful and validated entrance rituals might shape the first step in the ladder of social belonging which coming-of-age girls so desperately seek.

The modern western patriarchy does not welcome transformation for these girls. Transformation, by definition, includes some form of loss or change. The status quo of patriarchal script demands maintenance, not change, for women. "We would hardly expect that society itself would offer this rite of passage to women, who require it for the purpose of transforming the most fundamental norms of female identity" (Chernin, p. 167).

With no clear avenue for healthy passage, I took an unhealthy control route, as I believe many anorexic young girls do. Clinical, popular, and even feminist discourses on Anorexia seem to *help* anorexics by enabling them to regain weight and health without addressing the underlying psychological and familial issues, harmful discourses, and gendered inequalities. "The trouble with this *helping* is that it masks the sheer violence and disrespect embedded in the way in which anorexics are treated in psychiatric environments" (Saukko, p. 33).

My memoir exposes the disrespect that I personally experienced. Doctors forced me to gain weight and never asked why I had stopped eating. The emotional origins of my disorder were never considered or addressed. In a culture that values the body image, anorectics become conscious sculptors who may whittle away at their own flesh, creating a self-controlled image. Unconsciously, their self-starvation may also be an embodiment of a traditional rite of passage.

Transforming the perception of female identity in modern western society will require a deep cultural facelift as well as a celebration of that transformation. I hope to contribute to that reworking by having developed and implemented programs that empower women and girls to seek their truths and to tell their stories. These programs provide the space for group members to collaboratively develop empowered and transformational rituals.

## Notes

1 Habermas, 2015; Henderson et al., 2021; Holmes, 2016; Keel & Klump, 2003; Treasure & Campbell, 1994.

2 Ahmed, S. 2010; Bassoff, E. 1991; Bordo, S. 1988; Elza, C. 2018; Filipovic, J. 2017; Gilligan, C. 1982; hooks, b. 2004, 2015; McBride, H. et al. 2019; Rabinor, S. 1994; Ruti, M. 2014; Seid, R. 1994; Shisslak, C. & Craco, M. N. 1992; Solnit, R. 2017; Stoltenberg, J. 1990; Tolman, D. & Debold, E. 1994; Wolf, N. 1991; Woodman, M. 1993.

## References


Agostino, H., Burstein, B., Moubayed, D., Taddeo, D., Grady, R., Vyver, E., Dimitropoulos, G., Dominic, A., & Coelho, J. S. (2021). Trends in the incidence of new-onset anorexia nervosa and atypical anorexia nervosa among Youth During the COVID-19 Pandemic in Canada. *JAMA Network Open*, *4*(12), e2137395. https://doi-org.proxy.myunion.edu/10.1001/jamanetworkopen.2021.37395

Barrows, A. (2021, February). I wanted to love her not save her. *New York Times*.

Bordo, S. (1988). Anorexia nervosa: Psychopathology as crystallization of culture. In I. Diamond & L. Quinby (Eds.), In *Feminism and Foucault: Reflections on resistance.* Northeastern University Press.

Bordo, S. (1993). *Unbearable weight: Feminism, western culture and the body*. London University of California Press.

Chernin, K. (1985). *The hungry self: Women, eating and identity*. HarperCollins.

De Beauvoir, S. (1949). *The second sex.* Editions Gallimard.

De Beauvoir, S. (2011). *The second sex* (1st ed.). Vintage Books.

Holmes, S. (2016). Between feminism and anorexia: An autoethnography. *International Journal of Cultural Studies*, *19*(2), 193–207. https://doi.org.proxy.myunion.edu/10.1177/1367877914561831

Orbach, S. (1986). *Hunger strike: The anorectic's struggle as a metaphor for our age.* Faber & Faber.

Saukko, P. (2008). *The anorexic self: A personal and political analysis of a diagnostic discourse.* State University of New York Press.

Wolf, N. (1991). *The beauty myth: How images of beauty are used against women.* Morrow.

CHAPTER 5

# The Unholy Triumvirate—Art-Female-Nature

***Devalued Interventions***

> When writing to heal ourselves, we help others heal. In doing so, we can make our personal political.
>
> GIORGIO (2009, p. 149)

## 1 Introduction

The graduates of my master's program in Expressive Therapies were given the option to be *grandfathered* into the mental health system as Social Workers. At the time (1980) exercising this option, we were told, would benefit us professionally. Social work was science based, was more cognitive, was considered to be more male in its orientation and dissemination, thus more acceptable as treatment in the patriarchy. Expressive therapies, on the other hand, were arts and creativity based, less measurable, and deemed female in all aspects of their expression. I did not exercise the option to be grandfathered in. I felt that it would be cheating and, quite frankly, I did not want to be seen as a boring, eyebrow up, social worker. Those in my cohort that exercised the option to wear the socially acceptable mask of social worker, found jobs quickly. Sustained for me, was the inferior female posture, socially, academically, and now, professionally. I held to my conviction, however, to my truth, to my female way of working. Those hiding their truths behind the aegis of social worker, found jobs, but did not have the satisfaction and freedom as did I, to freely heal utilizing the arts. I understood that an Expressive therapist aspiring toward the top of the patriarchal pyramid must wear the acceptable persona. *Don't say anything artsy. Show the science behind the work you do. Only then will you be accepted academically or clinically. Pretend.*

Although all arts-based therapies have been devalued as female in western medicine, dance has perhaps been the lowest on the *totem pole*. Interesting that the image which I associate with the hierarchy, the totem pole, is an indigenous cultural ritual tool. Indigenous cultures, nature and earth based, revere

 | DOI:10.1163/9789004711051_006

the arts as healing modalities. Small wonder that their healing practices are disregarded in western medicine. Earth-nature-female-body: all irrelevant. The low status of dance is inextricably linked to its association with women and women's bodies. "Nevertheless, the exploration of dance and cultures and expressive anthropology reflects the centrality of dance and movement to many cultural rituals as well it's its productive role in culture. Dance therefore can produce insights into various aspects of different cultures" (Stinson quoted, Leavy, p. 182). I imagine that the cultures referenced by Leavy are indigenous, earth based, or matriarchal.

Dance Movement therapist and educator, Christine Caldwell traces this devaluing. She speak of DMT's (Dance Movement Therapy) disruption of the patriarchal bias in counseling:

> Criticism has been heaped onto traditional psychotherapies for being normed largely undead, straight, white males, and therefore inclining the field to look at healing through a patriarchal and sometimes misogynist lens, DMT can be seen as potentially disrupting this implicit patriarchal bias. The modalities emphasis on expressive movement and creativity, for instance, can be seen as generating more female centric-contributions to the overall understanding of how therapeutic change occurs. (Caldwell, 2016, p. 280)

We move our bodies before we are taught to speak. We hold in our bodies information about our lives that our conscious minds may suppress. The right side of our brain, the symbolic female side, the creative expressive side, sings and makes art. The left side, the symbolic male side, is analytic, it learns to speak. When we are distressed, when a traumatic event has occurred, the speaking side of the brain shuts down, thus *speechless terror*. However, the right side, the creative side is on board, ready to sing and to express. I have witnessed this in my work with traumatized children who are unable to express their narratives through words, but will sing about the event, dance it, write it, draw it. I have witnessed the power of what is called feminine therapy. It is important to understand this as we consider the value of arts-based interventions with children of trauma, specific to this book, anorexia. The feminine is the unseen, is the invisible: "Aspects of the invisible… which may not be actively remembered in the conscious mind, may emerge through dance" (Leavy, 2022, p. 189).

I have *waltzed* through talk therapy sessions with several clinicians over the years. Never once did my anorexia stand between us, asking to be heard. It was not until I began writing my memoirs, that her silenced voice began to leak out. With the assistance of music, visual prompts, and dance, I began to remember and reclaim my childhood trauma. Inspired by what I found, by what the expressive arts provided me with, I began to develop arts-based programs for girls and women. In this chapter, and specific to the book, I describe my integrated arts Teen Girl Empowerment workshop.

Provided here is a brief orientation to the memoir process with theme-based excerpts from my memoir.

## 2 Memoir

> The purpose of self-narrative is to extract meaning from experience rather than to depict experience exactly as it was lived. These narratives are not so much academic as they are existential, reflecting a desire to grasp or see the possibilities of meaning, which is what gives life its imaginative and poetic qualities… we narrate to make sense of experience over the course of time. (Boucher, 2000, p. 270)

My memoir explores, through my childhood experiences, both those factors that contributed to my anorexia, and those memories significant enough to present themselves to me today. Karr (2015) suggests that sensorial triggers help us to access memories: "Any single one will open up an *explosion of memories* associated with that sensorial catalyst. To develop voice… write your way into it from those explosions" (p. 71). Verbal prompts that trigger visual imagery provide me with access to my memories. I believe that I think in pictures; therefore, as I listen to music, I see visual forms; when I dance and move my body, I access equally, visual images into my mind's eye. From these prompts, I find my stories. Photo elicitation, as a modality, differs from verbal prompting as it produces a different kind of information; it evokes feelings, memories, and information. The parts of the brain that process visual information are, in evolutionary terms, older than the parts of the brain that process verbal information; therefore, visual images evoke deeper parts of human consciousness than words (Glaw et al., 2017).

Goldberg (2007) spoke of memoir as a form of survival in our patriarchal competitive culture:

> We are a dynamic country, fast paced ever onward. In the center of our speed, in the core of our forward movement, we are often confused and lonely. That's why we have turned so full heartedly to the memoir form. We have an intuition that it can save us. Writing is the act of reaching across the abyss of isolation to share and reflect. (p. XXI)

The narrative sequencing in my memoir, devoid of chronology, simulates the way memory is brought to consciousness. I weave between time periods inspired by visual, story and musical prompts. Goldberg (2007) points out that the mind recalls in a non-linear manner. We do not remember events chronologically. Memoir, she tells us, is "the study of memory, structured on the meandering way we remember. Essentially it is an examination of the zigzag nature of how our mind works" (p. xx).

> Experience is not linear, with a simple cause and effect, a beginning, and an end. It is rather a knot in a messy web; it is connected to a complexity of practices, histories, social structures, pure chances, and discourses that allude complete final mapping. (Saukko, 2008, p. 32)

My memoir sequences zig zag through time; I establish a chronological format which is based upon present day prompts and associations. Provided below are a few examples of themes associated with selected memoir snapshots.

## 3 My Memoir Themes and Memoir Excerpts

**Theme**: Pretense of belonging to be accepted into social groups.
**Memoir excerpts:** That I looked the part seemed important. I was not sure what the part was, but it was a part that I thought was necessary to take on. Mom reminded me that I should tell people, if they asked, that my last name was Strong. She did not want people to know that she had been married twice, so I could not tell my true last name which was Johnson.

Really, I did not belong in either group. Although we lived in the town as locals, we were nouveau locals having no heritage there. We never quite qualified for the country club set. Mom worked at obtaining entre into the club set, flashing her debutante and dressage credentials.

**Theme**: Lack of cultural rituals for transition into womanhood.
**Memoir excerpt:** The time to learn about becoming a woman, at least the physical woman, was sixth grade… Mom's response to my questions about getting my period was to give me a booklet, also published by Kotex. It was probably one she had been given as a teenager as the girls in the booklet were wearing clothes from the 40's and were engaged in activities that didn't seem modern… Mom had not made it clear what becoming a woman would involve. All that I understood at that time was what she showed by her actions. I was learning that being a woman meant telling a lot of lies and acting in a way that would

make me acceptable. My period revealed to me a distinction between truth and pretense, between what was inside and what was revealed.

**Theme:** Excessive collecting as result of anxious attachment for child of inconsistent mother: "An anxious attachment style is associated with a tendency to anthropomorphize comforting objects and an inability to tolerate distress, which in turn leads to excessive acquisition" (Norberg et al, 2018).
**Memoir excerpt:** Making babies came easy to her. In all, she had ten pregnancies. She lost a son before me, twins between Ann and Tommy, and another boy the year before Billy. As a mother to infants, she was the Queen. She seemed to lose interest when they learned to walk and talk, when they started to ask questions that demanded a different kind of attention.

**Theme:** Ambivalence toward mother:

The ambivalent child seems to be desperately trying to influence her mother. Many of them seem hooked by her haphazard, unpredictable style and the fact that she does come through on occasion. They pick up that she will respond sometimes, perhaps out of guilt, if they plead and make a big enough fuss (Karen, 1998, p. 221).

**Memoir excerpt:** Mostly my coming of age was being shaped by the conflicts between truths and lies. I wanted to be like Mom, but I was not sure which part of her presentation I wanted to mimic. She was beautiful, athletic, and musical. However, as I grew into consciousness (this did not happen until I was living away from home), I was able to stand back and see that the world she wanted everyone to see her in, was mostly make believe. It became harder and harder to know what was true and what she had made up. She had attempted to jinx us all, even her children….

Mom wanted me to be one of those pretty girls who was always front and center and that is why, for a while, she dressed me up to look like them. I know that I wanted to please her and sometimes, even to look like her.

## 4 Memoir as Autoethnographic

Autoethnography refers to writing about the personal and finding relevance to its relationship to culture. "An autoethnographic style posits the author is making a personal confession, as well as critically reflecting on her confession" (Saukko, p. 13). I suggest that the confession is expressed via the memoir and interpreted critically as a social statement. The interpretation may lie in the hands of the witness, the reader. Interpretation of any artistic expression is subjective. One could say that once expressed, the art no longer belongs to the artist. For each reader or witness, the art becomes their own. Each may superimpose personal meaning upon the art received. This reception and interpretation are what makes each story, dance, picture, musical composition collectively valuable to subjective audiences. When I write my stories, you will read them, resonate with or reject them according to your own life story. I rouse you to remember your own stories. However you receive and interpret mine, we are engaged and interacting in the process. The social potential for a group, for a society, might lie in valuing incorporation of individual stories into the collective:

> Speaking one's truth or truths through an autoethnographic lens, allows us to address the tensions between truths, whether personal or epistemological, in a political and hopeful act. It is political because it opens others' eyes to new realities of oppression and traumas; it is hopeful because it offers a chance for change. (Giorgio, 2009, p. 165)

## 5 Teen Girl Empowerment Workshop

### 5.1 *Inclusion of Identity and Ritual Work in Middle School Health Curriculum*

I have developed and launched a four-session art-based empowerment series for Middle School and High School girls; One such series has been incorporated into their health curriculum. The theme-based identity development series encourages self-reflection, with tools for accessing (in each respective theme-based session) Safety, Wisdom, Emotional Expression, and Resilience. My own coming-of-age identity confusion, brought to light by the process of writing my memoir, compelled me to create this workshop. I was hopeful that the workshop experience might help girls to experience the empowerment necessary to safely navigate their own identity development.

Readers are encouraged to engage, both personally and potentially as group leaders, in my described session activities. The format and sequencing are important to the fidelity of this program: (1) Opening circle ritual, (2) Central Activities, (3) Closure with Appreciations.[1] I have not included in this discussion, the specific music which I chose for each activity. However, the integration of music with movement and art activities is valuable.[2]

The initial pilot for this series was implemented with two age groups: High School combined grades 10 and 11 and Middle School grade 7. Later sessions were implemented with 8th and 6th grade girls respectively. Recruitment was conducted by school guidance counselors (who were trained in the protocol and who co-lead the groups with me). Parents were sent the following description along with the permission slips needed for participation. Informal evaluations followed which included these questions: (1) "Would you recommend this to your friends" and (2) "What from these four sessions do you take with you?"

## 6 Description of the Workshop for Parents and Teachers

Coming-of-age girls are bombarded with changes they may perceive to be out of their control. This time is ripe for identity confusion. This workshop provides a safe arts-based platform where girls might explore feeling associated with this coming of age, normalizing, and validating them all. It provides a safe space for exploring and participating in contemporary and traditional rites of passage into womanhood.[3]

These sessions offer multi-modal experiences within a consistent format. Included are gesture, movement, visual art, guided imagery, and journaling, all of which encourage the development or enhancement of individual and collective empowerment. Each session will be limited to 6 participants. No girl will be forced to engage in any activity. She will, however, benefit both emotionally and physiologically by simply attending and witnessing the session activities.

**Student Participants**

| | |
|---|---|
| High School Combined Grades 10 and 11 | January 2023 |
| Middle School Grade 7 | January 2023 |
| Middle School Grade 8 | April 2023 |
| Middle School Grade 6 | November 2023 |

**Structure and Content**

**Sessions 1: Grounding/Stability** **Earth Element Symbology**

**Tools needed:**

Music
Parachute
Ball/Talking Stick
Rocks
Silks
Fabric markers

## 7 Opening Circle Ritual

*Begin the session by discussing confidentiality. The importance of journal writing after each experiential activity is discussed. Additionally, I mention that each session has a Nature symbolic theme. The first, grounding and stability is represented by "earth."*

The circle is the most ancient symbol, the architecture of containment, is expressive of equality and completion, is the sun and the earth in eternal motion, is the roundness of pregnancy, of vessels, is the home that represents stability. It encloses emptiness. When we leave the center of a movement (dance) circle empty and focus our collective attention toward this unmoved stillness, we find within ourselves the calm of this center. In spite of the chaos which exists outside the circle, we are assured the potential, with our ability to focus on stillness. By simply holding hands to create a physical circle, the experience of relationship is transformed from "self and other" to "self as part of a greater whole." As girls gather together in circles, their individual strengths and beauties are affirmed; This affirmation makes it possible to rebuild the social communities which conflict has destroyed.

1. Opening Ritual
    a. Sitting Intro: *Name and Story* (pass around talking stick)
    Each student will tell their name and will provide an associative narrative. This may be as simple as where their name originated or a nick name that they prefer. Often students will share the cultural meaning of their name.
    b. Gesture dance in circle (bring breath into body, calm, connection)
        1. Begin with hands placed upon the heart-Arms open above, eyes and palms facing up
        2. Hands placed back upon heart
        3. Arms gesture as if gathering the whole circle to that person
        4. Hands again placed upon heart
        5. Arms extend outward and forward with palms facing upward
        6. Palms turn downward as hands slowly move to touch the ground

Hands placed back upon heart: *vocalize* to music provided:

(1) *"Open to sky"* (2) *"Light to your heart"* (3) *" To your friends"* (4) *"Back to your heart"* (5) *"Offering friendship"* (6) *"and share with the earth"*[4]

2. Central Activities
   a. Parachute collective activity sitting and standing: Group member hold the (12 foot) parachute's edge engaging in the following collective movements: Pull-Rest and Circling. The parachute is moved collectively providing a non-intimate yet empowering experience.
   b. Rock Sculpture: Self Statement and Collective Engagement
   This exercise allows participants to experience with Nature symbolism, both personal and group attachment experiences.
      1. Each participant is instructed to choose 8 from collection of rocks brought by the interventionist.
      2. In silence and solitude, they will create a personal sculpture from their chosen rocks (20 min).
      3. Students are asked to consider what meaning (persons, places, ideas) may be associated with their chosen rocks (this is a self-statement).
      4. Each participant chooses 3 of the 8 rocks, bringing them to the group circle. Each takes a turn with the goal being the creation of a group sculpture. The only rules/guidelines are: 1) One person at a time, 2) Do not move another's object, and 3) witness silently each person's addition.
   c. Safe Place Activity (Safe Covers): Each student is provided with a white silk 21" scarf and encouraged to draw upon it an image (person, place, symbol), color or word that they associate with: safety or love. This is done in silence and sharing will follow. Students may share verbally or simply by showing their safe cover.[5]
3. Closure

**Appreciations**: Students are encouraged to share some aspect of the group which they have appreciated or enjoyed today. This may be: Spoken, gestured, or considered silently.

**Session 2: Wisdom/Spirit** **Air Element Symbology**

**Tools needed:**

Music,

Parachute

Crapas

Paper/journals
Peacock feathers
Long scarves

1. Opening Circle Ritual
    a. Gesture Dance (think of Question you have about present, past or future life challenge: to be accessed in Animal Ally Ex)[6]
    b. Standing Circle: Hold parachute at periphery and verbalize as move these directives: "Down-Up-Under and Away."
    c. Circle Wind Runs without Parachute: Dropping the parachute to the floor, students are guided to move to the center as if pushed by the wind, then withdraw back to starting place as if pulled backward by the wind. This encourages the experience of moving organically as one drawn forward and backward by the wind (associated with one's own breath which moves each individual)
2. Central Activities Experiences
    a. Guided Meditation to Find Animal Guide:
        1. Envision blue dot,inhale:dot expands to become blue sky
        2. Fill sky w/ landscape: rainforest, jungle, plain, desert, mt, water place
        3. Imagine yourself in the lansdscape
        4. Sounds?smells?colors?time of day?
        5. Let animal enter landscape. Whatv does it looks likes? Sounds? feel?
        6. Let self transform into animal…explore movements
        7. Envision Animal and Move as, find sounds
        8. *Draw Pix write words associated w/ animal; circle 4 words-use to write a poem*

Process/Sharing in group circle: How will your guide be able to help me with roadblocks/journey[7,8]

    b. Air/Breath work:
    Air: Feather and scarf Balancing (calming, serotonin releasing)\
    Integration of breath with movement via visual/tactile focus; Carry scarf in outstretched arms moving forward rocking back and forth, focusing upon scarf in arms.
    And/or
    Balance Peacock feather in one hand focusing upon eye of feather. Students may move the feather from one hand top another and later try passing a feather between two students.

3. Closure
Make a sound that represents your appreciation today.

**Session 3: Emotion/Expression/Vocalize** **Water Element Symbology**

**Tools needed:**
Music,
Parachute
Crapas
Paper/journals
Long scarves

**Suggested prompts for this sessions** WATER; all emotions: struggle-rage-love-death-birth

DA VINCI on water
Water is the driver of nature: If you throw a stone in a pond. The waves which strike against the shores are thrown back toward the spot where the stone struck; and on meeting other waves they never intercept each other's course. In a small pond one and the same stroke gives birth to many motions of advance and recoil.

1. Opening Ritual
    a. Gesture Dance (as before adding vocal toning: "EE-Oh-Ah-OH"[9]
    b. Parachute Circle add: Fountain/Chalice Collective Ritual: To lyrical 4/4 music group scoops "water from individual water source at feet and carries together to shared rhythm, the collective waters which, chalice like, create fountain at center ...followed by wind run circle (slow to fast movement) Music
2. Central Activities
    a. Spiral Dance: Each with long scarf spiral around room with image of water embodied: group leader gives verbal prompts: "rain-river-waterfall-ocean-cloud-storm cloud,etc")
    b. Water Wheel: Draw self at center of ocean (starfish). All other positive relationships are drawn as symbolic water creatures (give examples: support-protect-love-respect). This is a variation upon the Psychometric "Social Atom"[10]
    c. Yes/No: Two lines stand opposite one another and vocalize.
    d. Mirror/Mirror: Students are asked to imagine looking into a familiar mirror.
    What does the mirror say? Write down or draw what is reflected back to you.
    Does it say what you would like it to say or reflect how you feel about yourself?
    If the mirror was a person telling you what it does, who would that person be?

Do you have anything that you'd like to say back to that mirror/ person?[11,12]

3. Closure

Appreciations: Strike a pose or make a gesture that reflects how you would like people to see you. Group reflects each individual's pose to amplify and validate the positive expression,.

**Session 4: Strength/Energy/Resilience Fire Element Symbology**

**Session Prompt:** FIRE is of the spirit. PROMETHEUS gave us fire (new things rising must be faced

Give self permission to be pierced by light (light makes fire)

Make space in self for light to come in.

**Tools needed:**

Music,
Parachute
Crapas
Paper/journals
Long scarves (red)
Long paper for group strength drawing
Something symbolic of torches for relay

1. Opening Ritual
   a. Gesture Dance (complete with toning)
   b. Add to Parachute activity:
      *Trust in Self/Group: Relationship Progression*
      This is an exercise that allows each participant to trust the group and a partner, to support his/her weight, and to feel the benefits of surrender/support.
      1. The whole group holds on to the edges of the open parachute (Intermediary object).
      2. Rhythmically the sing and move to this pattern: *Pull and Rest* (Pulling, they are supported by the group pulling the parachute. (Rest: they return to self-support)
      3. The group exercise repeats without the parachute, with participants holding each other at elbow level.
      4. The elbow held experience may be done in dyads.
2. Central Activities
   a. Fire Circle: Create Collective Energy:
      With something symbolic of fire in center of the circle (candle, red scarf), the students create a circle around the center, gaze into

it, with arms open and palms facing inward, pulse forward and back,with long exhales as pulse forward.

b. Run the Gauntlet: Imagine the other students who are place between you and a goal are the *obstacles* to achieving that goal. Each takes a turn running through the *obstacles*. Students in the role of *obstacles* do not touch or aggress upon the soloist, rather hold their hands up and move their bodies in a manner that embodies *obstacle*. Each gets a turn to run through the gauntlet.[13]

c. Torch Relay: *Two groups pass torch in relay race (2 tied silk scarf knotted)*[14]

d. Group Strength Drawing: Group assembles together around a 6-foot length of paper. One participant volunteers to lie down on the paper and have their body outline traced by the rest of the group. To avoid association with a dead body tracing, I refer to the body outlined as a *shape*. After the outline is complete the volunteer may stand up and in silence all participants are asked to focus on the outline of the *shape* and to think about where they feel safety and strength in their body. Music is now started and participants dance around the tracing in a circle. When the music is stopped participants may kneel down and begin drawing inside and outside the *shape* where they feel their safety and strength may be. This will repeat for 5 or 6 rounds until the body tracing is full or completed. Each group shares as they sit around the drawing and then the large group may walk around and view all the small group drawings. Music may be played during this time.

3. Closure

Final Appreciations: Students are asked to consider "What Do You Take with You from this Experience?": (Can shut eyes and let an image come-embody and have group reflect). Final journal entries follow. After this session students take their journals home with encouragement to continue writing or drawing their thoughts.

## 8 My Observations from Pilot Groups

What I understood to be clear goals and distinctions between the two groups were the following: The 7th graders never slowed down to take a breath and so we worked with them on activities that would bring the full range of breathing (inhale and exhale cycle) into the bodies through the moving activities that were slow and calming. This group did very well with moments of stillness and slow moving. It appears that the nature of their school schedule with few breaks in between classes certainly magnified that tendency to never slow down and or to rest in between activities and movements. We would continue to work on this slowing down while encouraging the maintenance of their joyful expression and spontaneity.

For the older girls, the 10th and 11th graders, the major goal as I saw it, was to help them find comfort in being witnessed by others. Activities in which they were contemplative, creative or solitary seemed to be the most comfortable for them all. Their verbal sharing was sophisticated and deep, but they were unable to find comfort with moving their bodies or stepping outside their comfort level in the presence of others. I would like to work with them on experiencing witnessing as supportive rather than judgmental. This may take another round of four sessions.

The theme of "Belonging" was clearly present for both age groups. I posit that for the younger girls, in their desire to understand who they are and how they fit into their peer group, they mimicked the powerful peer leaders and were reticent to present as differing from this model. This appeared significantly for girls who were ethnically or physically different. Acting silly appeared to be the comfortable default presentation. For the older girls this desire to belong was amplified. It appeared that the acceptable social norm had already been established (culturally, politically) and these girls will not veer from any expression that might distinguish them from this norm. This rigid adherence truncated their willingness to explore their amazing creative differences. Our culture tells us that diversity is not valued. In some cases, the presentation of differences is seen as a punishable offense. In our world girls are taught that to advance socially and financially, they must mimic the male prototype. The media female ideal contradicts this male prototype. So, who is she to be, this budding identity? Act like a man but look like the exaggeration of femininity? Which one will prevail?

## Notes

1 The circle is the most ancient symbol, the architecture of containment, is expressive of equality and completion, is the sun and the earth in eternal motion, is the roundness of pregnancy, of vessels, is the home that represents stability. It encloses emptiness. When we leave the center of a movement (dance) circle empty and focus our collective attention toward this unmoved stillness, we find within ourselves the calm of this center. In spite of the chaos which exists outside the circle, we are assured the potential, with our ability to focus, on

stillness. By simply holding hands to create a physical circle, the experience of relationship is transformed from "self and other" to "self as part of a greater whole." As girls gather together in circles, their individual strengths and beauties are affirmed; This affirmation makes it possible to rebuild the social communities which conflict has destroyed.

2 Music creates an acoustic container which encourages the sense of safety and minimizes the perception of being alone.

3 I know that teens are hungry for such rituals. As an example: my son Dylan was staged to graduate from college in May of 2020. Because of the Covid pandemic, his last two months of school were virtual, and his graduation ceremony was cancelled. He and his classmates were given the option to have a virtual graduation the following year. They chose not to exercise this option and rather told the administration: "We will wait until we can have a live ceremony with caps and gowns and the pomp and circumstance." His school, Pitzer College, respected the wishes of these students who will participate in this rite of passage ritual, two years later, in May 2022. This profoundly affected me. I understood that the need for ritual goes beyond my contemporaries. I heard increasingly that high school students, limited to virtual interaction, had chosen to create their own rituals and ceremonies. Some teachers had listened to their voices and have validated their wishes. The need to have these young voices heard and responded to shapes my recommendation for creating the space for their art and rituals, both individual and collective to emerge.

4 *Vocalization: 7th:* These girls especially love vocalizing with the prompt to make it as big and loud as you can they have no problem with this activity and seem to enjoy the familiarity of having it repeat each time in exactly the same way. 10/11: These older girls were reticent to vocalize, looking around to see what peers were doing.

5 *Safe covers:* Here students were focused and engaged/They were contemplative rather than expressive to group. Generally, they were reticent to say anything that made them present as different or not belonging. I discussed the value of diversity in nature and how different and unique all of them are yet have much in common. All the same would be boring. Encouragement to journal what they have discovered and feel uncomfortable sharing verbally with the group.

6 Safe place in circle established and sustained: Each girl sat in the same spot in the circle each week.

7 Another Dance Therapist created a similar curriculum and. Reflected: "Their verbal responses became the catalyst for embodied movement of emotion as perceived by each individual participant. As the characters interacted with each other, the participants began to change their movements in order to stand their ground, demonstrate the emotion more fully, or otherwise embody their understanding of the emotion from the safe position of imaginative play. During this exercise, the author observed the formation of embodied narratives at both individual and group levels. Through their unique ways of dancing and moving, the participants demonstrated a personal relationship to each emotion. Additionally, as they moved in relationship to each other, they revealed their relationship to the embodiment of emotion in another person" (Thomas, p.187) Anna Halperin suggested experiential.

8 Here, my students seemed self-conscious, walking rather than moving to the music or as the animal envisioned, moving only their arms in a restricted manner (from elbow rather than thorax) flying or swimming. It appears that when cued to move as an ensemble rather than free form, they were more able to move with full body expression.

9 Vocal toning with vowel sounds energize specific parts of the spine and allow for full breath cycle as chant

10 *Water wheel:* The students were very engaged and excited about sharing how each of the sea creatures was representative of the person in their life that they were symbolizing. Much

information was revealed regarding very different family configurations and emotions and dynamics in their respective families.

11 *Time as mirror:* I think of the many physical mirrors that I have gazed into over the passage of my life. In particular, I remember a mirror that was in my childhood home. I gazed into it every day during my youth and found myself returning to it as a point of reference, a barometer of sorts, in my adult life. Gazing into it, I would see my reflection of my current self, in her embodied aging shell. This changing shell was defined by the mirror which was a constant, a mirror from my youth that projected who my changing shell self was and how she would be known. And, every person and place that we have a relationship with provides us with a different mirror. Therefore, we have a diversity of mirrors, all which contribute to our identity. Understanding that there are a multitude of projections, from us to them, and they to us, should be illuminating. As we consider that there is more than binarism, is it not helpful to consider this multitude of mirrors? Over time, expanding the many roles we play, all of which contribute rather than compete within us. Might this paradigm not translate to the whole of social exchange and identity?

12 *Mirror Experience:* Much time was spent on journaling for this activity. In sharing, students were thoughtful and curious about the difference between how they see themselves based on social mandates and superficial perception and how the person that loves and respects them see something different. I spent some time discussing how people are like mirrors and we often are around people that judge us or look at us in a negative way and that affects how we see ourselves. Sometimes we can't avoid those people but we can be empowered to seek out and balance that negativity with being around people that love and respect us.

13 *Gauntlet:* This activity which is very aerobic seem to be popular. The girls seemed to most enjoy being the obstacles and true to their expression in other sessions were less willing to get out there and be the individual moving towards her goal. With prompting everybody did take on that role. It seemed that when the other students were encouraging each individual, they were more willing to get up there and move through the obstacles.

14 *Relay Race:* This was the most popular moving activity so far for this group. I think that it was because there was a challenge that was based on engagement with each other and they were able to focus on the torch rather than their bodies moving. Focusing upon an intermediary object assists those reticent to move while being witnessed to meet the goal of moving.

## References

Boucher, A. P. (2000) Criteria against ourselves. *Qualitative Inquiry, 6*, 266–272.

Caldwell, C., & Leighton, L. (October, 2016). Dance/Movement therapy, women's rights, and feminism: The first 50 years. *American Journal of Dance Therapy, 38*, 279–284.

Giorgio, G. (2009). Traumatic truths and the gift of telling. *Qualitative Inquiry, 15*(1), 149–167.

Glaw, X., Inder, K., Kable, A., & Hazelton, M. (2017). Visual methodologies in qualitative research: Autophotography and photo elicitation applied to mental health research. *International Journal of Qualitative Methods, 16*(1–8). Sage Publications.

Goldberg, N. (2007). *Old friend from far away: The practice of writing memoir*. Simon & Schuster.

Karr, M. (2015). *The art of memoir.* HarperCollins Publishers.
Leavy, P. (2009). *Method meets art: Arts-based research practice.* Guildford.
Saukko, P. (2008). *The anorexic self: A personal and political analysis of a diagnostic discourse.* State University of New York Press.

CONCLUSION

# We Speak

> In the middle of winter, I at last discovered that there was in me an invincible summer.
>
> CAMUS, RETOUR À TIPASA

∴

## ME

When I was fourteen, I stopped eating, and no one asked me why. When I was thirty-eight, no one had ever thrown me a surprise birthday party. I decided to throw one for myself. Both scenarios made me feel invisible, unnoticed, and unimportant. This was my sense of self for most of my life. I had been waiting to be acknowledged. Acting for myself rather than waiting to be acted upon would have taken courage in my youth. Taking action, as I did in both cases as an adult, was catalyzed not by courage, but rather by exasperation. I took the bull by the horns and made what had been denied to me by others, happen.

It took me a very long time to feel the competence necessary to ask for, or to take something, for myself. I believed that if I had been asked why I had stopped eating when I was fourteen, my life would have been different. The overwhelming lack of esteem that I felt as a teenager impacted all my consequent relationships, romantic, familial, and professional. Mackenzie (1991) of anorexics' narratives, states: "One overwhelming concern I have heard is the need to strive for enough self-respect to feel entitled to form relationships with others in society. Such self-esteem is to be achieved through restrained eating" (p. 408). The almost fatal combination of forced pretense and lack of esteem, as I hope my memoirs reflect, truncated my identity development.

## US

This book, I am hopeful, brings to light the importance of listening to each girl. When truly listened to, she might begin to listen to herself. She might find value in what she has forgotten to hear. She is worthy of your time and attention. Her

 | DOI:10.1163/9789004711051_007

story *really* matters. Her story is like no other story. And by giving her your greatest gift, your time, you may find that her story teaches you something new. You may find yourself loving this new story. And there are many stories, each unique and worthy of your attention. Time and love given to each new bud will allow our social and global gardens to grow.

In the end, it is the responsibility of all humans to challenge and change the Patriarchy. Time and love have lost their value. Speed and aggression reign sovereign here. In his race we all lose momentum, and no one can really win. Sisyphus. Alone, fearful, ashamed, devalued, lost. Let us slow down and listen to, not only the girls, but to each other. The tortoise, she is silent, slow, and steady. Let us be like the tortoise and we might transform the race into a celebratory welcome into a new harmonious world.

## Reference

Mackenzie, M. (1991, December). Review of fasting girls: The emergence of anorexia nervosa as a modern disease by Joan Jacobs Brumberg: Fasting Girls: The surprising history of anorexia nervosa. *Medical Anthropology Quarterly, 5*(4), 406–410.

# Subject Index

# Name Index

www.ingramcontent.com/pod-product-compliance
Lightning Source LLC
Chambersburg PA
CBHW071344230926
51846CB00002B/444

* 9 7 8 9 0 0 4 7 1 1 0 3 7 *